'The puppet is a tool – a weapon to transform the subconscious, to stir the emotions and to re-connect our memory. I understand this concept, and as Karrie discusses, it really works. I have worked all my life in using the puppet to break down barriers and get messages across to the public throughout the world. Be it with AIDS education, democracy and corruption education or creativity and communication in schools, universities or the corporate world, the results are always the same. The puppet or inanimate object has an innate power to communicate on a "soul level". A simple movement by an inanimate object fascinates us and can move us to tears without necessarily saying a word. Karrie puts it very aptly: we connect in the moment of "now".'

– *Gary Friedman, Gary Friedman Productions, CEO Corporate Creatures, and editor of www.puppetrynews.com*

'Triumph over adversity is something that is often praised, but this book shows us how to get so much more. Creating joy where there was despair is something so powerful as to seem miraculous. Karrie Marshall shows us the great value of using puppetry in care settings to achieve just that and then gives us the tools to do it for ourselves. Powerful, inspiring and empowering.'

– *Keith Walker, Policy Officer – Health Improvement, Highland Council, Choose Life Highland Coordinator*

'Calmly and lucidly, Karrie Marshall tells extraordinary stories of the positive impact which just one art form – puppetry – can have in one crucial and highly emotive field of healthcare: dementia. In doing so she also reminds us that we've not yet grasped the full power of the arts to change lives.'

– *Robert Livingstone, Director of HI~Arts, promoting the arts in the Highlands and Islands of Scotland*

'This book provides an excellent justification for the use of art, and more specifically puppetry, as a way of connecting with people with dementia who might otherwise have difficulties maintaining social interaction. Karrie Marshall has obviously researched her subject thoroughly and this book will be of use to anyone who has contact with people with dementia whether they be activity coordinators in

care homes, formal carers or relatives. It seeks to introduce novel ways of enhancing the quality of life for people with dementia, at whatever stage they are in the condition.'

– Dr Samantha Murphy, lecturer and Chair of the Open
University module on Death and Dying, and module author on
forthcoming Open University module on Dementia Care

'With her innovative, creative approach, founded on years of experience, mixed with compassion, humour and boundless enthusiasm, Karrie builds beautiful bridges of hope, empowerment and inspiration for clients, relatives and staff alike.'

– Jo Munroe, Project Worker (social care)

Puppetry in Dementia Care

Connecting through Creativity and Joy

Karrie Marshall

Jessica Kingsley *Publishers*
London and Philadelphia

The 'You Are my Sunshine' lyrics on p.127 are reproduced with kind permission from Peer International Corporation. Copyright © Peer International Corporation 1940.

First published in 2013
by Jessica Kingsley Publishers
116 Pentonville Road
London N1 9JB, UK
and
400 Market Street, Suite 400
Philadelphia, PA 19106, USA

www.jkp.com

Library of Congress Cataloging in Publication Data
Marshall, Karrie.
Puppetry in dementia care : connecting through creativity and joy / Karrie Marshall.
  pages cm
Includes bibliographical references and index.
ISBN 978-1-84905-392-1 (alk. paper)
1. Dementia--Patients--Care. 2. Puppets--Therapeutic use. 3. Arts--Therapeutic use. I. Title.
RC521.M373 2013
616.89'1656--dc23
                2013004883

British Library Cataloguing in Publication Data
A CIP catalog record for this book is available from the British Library

ISBN 978 1 84905 392 1
eISBN 978 0 85700 848 0

Printed and bound in Great Britain by Bell & Bain Ltd, Glasgow

And the children in the apple-tree
Not known, because not looked for
But heard, half-heard, in the stillness
Between two waves of the sea.
('Little Gidding V', by T.S. Eliot 1942)

We're made of stars in the night
Shine on invincible.
(Song lyrics 'My Memory is Like a Dolphin',
K. Marshall 2012)

Contents

Acknowledgements

Thank you to everyone who gave their time, energy and support for my creative programmes over the past ten years. I am profoundly grateful to each person in this book, for sharing stories, wisdom and humour.

For your readiness to make creative connections that inspire other people, thank you Margaret and John Vernal, Jimpy Mendham, Murdo Fraser, June Webb, Eva MacLennan, Dick Mardon, Ana-Maria Pearson, Sandra, Margaret, Mr and Mrs Hastings, Mr and Mrs Pryde, June Ross and many more individuals whose names remain safe in my heart, and whose magical puppets live on.

For your willingness to trust the process, share insights, difficulties and laughter, my appreciation goes to every family and staff member and care home connected with this work.

Thank you to Wendy Mumford for your letters saying 'Write the book!'; to my husband Chris King for your loving support and essential cups of tea; Chris Brotherston for your enthusiasm and Robert Livingston for your encouragement. Thanks to my sister Jo Munroe for knowing this was possible, my brother Nigel for being the first person to buy this book and my brother Mick for cheering me on.

Finally, my grateful thanks to Christine Firth, the copy editor, for helping me through the process and keeping me on track!

Introduction

The Man with a Kitten in His Pocket

David found it difficult to spend much time with his mum. She did not recognise him, and David did not understand her broken sentences. They sat in awkwardness. Helen's anxious glances at her son, who was now a stranger, bore more heavily on him with each visit. He checked his watch, waiting for a reasonable amount of time to pass before leaving.

In the past he had brought news and photographs of his family. Together they would delight in the children's achievements at school, or recall recent happy birthdays, holidays, and Christmas celebrations. They would crack open a bottle of lemonade and eat favourite biscuits. Visiting had a sense of purpose. David knew what to do and Helen enjoyed herself too.

The loss of memory gradually reached the faces in the photographs, and then David himself. They still shared the biscuits, but even this seemed a little clumsy...out of context. The care home provided reminiscence therapy while checks were made for other possible underlying causes of memory loss and confusion.

David noticed his mum was doing her best to keep up the appearance of remembering, but this was a strain for her. Anxiety-reducing medication was prescribed for the severe bouts of nervousness that sometimes accompanied the confusion. David did not know how to be with her any more.

He did not want to give up seeing her, and yet he was struggling to see what benefit there could be for his mum. Helen always seemed a little shocked when he sat in the chair next to her, so he had found himself sitting a little further away, hoping she might feel more relaxed. Helen politely nodded, and her son nodded back. There was little communication.

It was a kitten puppet that changed things. The puppeteers worked with Helen. She seemed to like all the puppets, and fleetingly joined in with their songs or banter. But it was the kitten in a handbag that really made the difference. As soon as Helen noticed the kitten glove puppet, she welcomed it with all the love and delight in the world. Her voice was clear and her words were about beauty and joy.

The kitten became her constant companion. She sang to it, held it, kissed it, stroked it, and protected it. During one session, the puppeteers brought another kitten puppet to meet hers. Helen was thrilled. The kittens played together. Over subsequent weeks Helen had conversations about things kittens do. (The list is endless!) She described the kitten climbing up the curtains, or coming home with muddy paws.

David learned that he could also connect with his mum through the puppet. He kept one in his pocket for visiting. Together, and for the next two years, Helen and her son shared kitten stories. The visits regained a sense of purpose. They connected in the world of puppetry, where there is no pressure to remember anyone.

This is a book about possibilities. It is dedicated to all the people who experienced isolation because we did not know any better – and now we do. Knowing better comes from believing that things can be different. A person in the late stages of dementia may seem lost to the world, but what if there is another perspective? What if we can connect beyond words and memory? What if we can even find genuine joyfulness? Have a great laugh? Share significant moments?

Then we would not be filled with fear and despair. We would have a sense of hope for all the carers and cared for. This book aims to inspire creative and meaningful ways of connecting with people, whose memory, words and relationships are affected by conditions, such as dementia. My work is with adults who have recently been diagnosed with dementia as well as people experiencing mid and late stage dementia symptoms.

Over the years I have found common issues experienced by staff in care homes and carers at home, which affect the quality of life of the people they care for. Some issues are to do with perspective or cultural views about dementia. In the media and at conferences we have heard alarming phrases about dementia: 'terrible epidemic'; 'devastating'; 'world time bomb'; 'veritable health plague'; 'most feared disease'; 'dreadful suffering'; 'cruel and tragic disease'.[1]

And people with dementia say, 'Love us for who we are.' It is difficult for everyone concerned when the mass response to dementia is fear. It is a sensitive and profoundly moving subject. None of us likes to consider losing our identity or finding ourselves in a world that is unfamiliar, with people we do not recognise. There is a rise in the number of people diagnosed with dementia, which is in correlation to the increasing population age, but we must be clear that dementia is not an inevitable part of ageing, and not everyone experiences the same symptoms. What we need therefore is hope and information, ideas and practical help, and even the slightest possibility of joyfulness.

More people are realising that there are ways in which they can create positive connections. Sometimes lack of confidence or uncertainty about what to do is all that stands in the way of powerful contact. I have met carers (at home and in care homes) who describe the distancing that occurs as communication becomes more awkward. Exclusion and isolation increase. It does not have to be this way.

We all do the best we can with what we know; and what we know is often affected by how we feel. The better we feel, the more open we are to other perspectives. This book offers stories of love and joy. It is full of examples of human strength and capacity. People may have been written off in the past, but here we see their wonderful gifts, or their humour and sensitivities.

The book explains the importance of creative connections. I use puppetry to express ideas and communicate experiences with adults in education; adults in care work; adults using mental health services and people using care services in general. I also work with adults with fronto-temporal lobe dementia (FTD), Alzheimer's disease, vascular dementia and dementia with Lewy bodies (DLB), and with people who experience memory loss and confusion, but who have not been diagnosed with dementia.

As we explore the fascinating medium of puppetry, you will see how the form yields fascinating results. Other art forms are included, as puppetry encompasses many genres. Underlying care principles increase the quality of the work and experiences for people living with dementia. Respect for individuality, compassion, listening, empathy, creativity, support and a sense of possibility are key elements.

Each chapter begins with a story about puppetry with people who had experienced isolation. The stories are occasionally an amalgamation of two people's experiences, or the genders and names have been changed. This is to protect the identity of individuals with whom we work, unless otherwise desired by the person and their family or staff.

There are practical activities, hints and tips throughout the book. Some exercises can be undertaken quickly. Other activities are designed as programmes, which are done in stages. This is the way we usually work – building activities over a few sessions, alongside single-stage events. The creative process is extremely valuable, so we explore ways to mark genuine success, even if the main task is incomplete.

Creativity is all-inclusive. There is no right or wrong about it. Sometimes people are concerned that they cannot draw, so they feel they are not creative. Yet they may have planned a garden or concocted a meal. At some point many of us have created mountains out of molehills, made a card, painted a wall, told a spur of the moment joke, invented a name, made up lyrics, created a scrapbook or arranged objects in a particular formation on a shelf.

Creativity can be found in ordinary domestic life as well as in the extraordinary world of arts, crafts and performance. This book gives guidance on the making and using of puppets. But first I want to look briefly at the role of creativity in health care.

A case for creativity in care

It is exciting to see all the research showing links between creativity and mental well-being. Hannemann (2006) explains that creative activity has been shown to reduce depression and isolation. There is a clear change in people during the puppetry sessions. Sometimes individuals begin low in mood or very tired. But they become more alert and their eyes shine. A host of factors contribute to this, as we explore later.

Activity coordinators, occupational therapists and other professionals see the positive impact of their work, particularly with people who can actively participate. Engagement in activities can improve quality of life in social, emotional, intellectual and physical areas. It is something all carers can do, in a variety of ways, from the simple to the complex, depending on energy and time available. People experiencing late stages of brain disease can still connect if we create the right environments for them.

Cohen (2006a) ran creativity and ageing studies. His findings show that we are capable of creative expression throughout our entire life cycles. Our creativity and imagination do not seem to reduce at the same rate as memory or language. This explains why connecting through creativity rather than through words alone is so important. Some relatives tell us they notice an increase in creativity as dementia progresses, but it may be that as other skills or functions 'fall away', the imagination and creativity are more noticeable.

There is not an agreed definitive location in the brain for creativity. Perhaps, like consciousness and intuition, it is not tied to a place. Speech, motor skills, vision and hearing all have their locations in the brain, but even these may have the potential to move. Following a stroke, patients may improve as a result of the brain's plasticity, which is the ability of undamaged brain tissue to take over functions previously handled by a part that was damaged (Burkman 1998).

Miller conducted research into how the brain is affected by degenerative diseases such as Alzheimer's. He notes that even though our brains age, it does not diminish our ability to create: 'As people [with dementia] lose the ability to name, to conceptualise what things are, they are forced into much more visual ways of thinking about the world' (Miller 2004).

As words become confused or the memory shifts take place, we all have an opportunity to engage with people through creative practice. Creativity is an essential part of being human. It is how we get our ideas and innovations; how we solve problems and imagine our futures. And it is how we make things and express ourselves. Patricia Baines (2007), an Australian art therapist, writes about the sense of awe when watching a person with dementia paint or write, because regardless of memory loss, the person is expressing and revealing a unique identity: 'The very process of being a creator empowers, by allowing for a flow of energy and life. It makes well' (Baines 2007, p.5).

Coming from a family of carers and artists (and philosophers), it has always seemed natural for me to marry creativity and care work. Care may include the arts as part of a holistic treatment (arts in health), or art may be used as a therapy in itself (art therapy). While my interest spans both areas, I find myself drawn to arts as a part of holistic caring – arts as something in which we can all participate in numerous ways. Understanding of the value of creative practice has been known for generations.

Medical superintendents inspected asylums in the 1800s and recorded their observations and suggestions for improvements. Bible readings, storytelling, drawing, sewing, dancing and annual concerts were encouraged. A promoter of activities for mental and physical well-being was the medical officer of Crichton Royal Institution, Scotland, W.A.F. Browne. In the 1830s, he advocated gardens, farms, occupation and a range of activities including art, drama, music, readings and games (Browne 1976).

The term 'art therapy' came in 1942, when Adrian Hill practised art while recovering from tuberculosis (cited by Hogan 2001). He was later employed as a therapist and developed art therapy through the British Red Cross society and the National Association for the Prevention of Tuberculosis. The National Health Service (NHS) took on artists informally. Now there are dedicated art psychotherapy university courses. State registration is required before practising as an art therapist. The job includes enabling individuals to work through their emotions about their illness or conditions.

Arts in health can have a social function. It was an important part of life in the long stay hospitals. Staff and relatives of people living there made costumes and attended the annual concerts and pantomimes. These participative arts were often considered the highlight of the year. As many people as possible would be included. It was an opportunity to shine; to be important and break out of the everyday routines. The therapeutic gains of being a part of this creative experience are still remembered by staff and former patients.

The benefits of creativity in care have regularly been identified through qualitative evaluations. This often takes the form of people expressing how arts and art activities have affected them. My own observations and experiences in care homes are often recorded on film. The advantages of creative activity repeatedly show increased self-esteem and improved quality of life. There are many other anecdotal benefits, such as pride in personal achievements; reduction in stress; increase in self-expression and communication; enhanced spirituality; openness; enjoyment; and skill development.

Arts as part of the physical and aesthetic environment is important too. Hospitals now incorporate professional art, design and architecture in their refurbishments to enhance the patient experience. Research in the 1970s by Roger Ulrich showed that people recovered more quickly from surgery when they had views of landscape and trees (cited by Miles 1994). How simple it is for us to hang a picture of beauty in clear sight to help someone feel better.

People who are used to creative practice are probably familiar with the accompanying deep sense of peace. This might not be expected with people in the mid to late stages of dementia, whose focus and concentration spans are so variable. But we found the creative peace was there just the same as for any other group of people. Years have shown us that creativity has its own magic. People who engage seem to experience the creative silence. It comes when they are the makers, the explorers, the poets or painters, the puppeteers or the observers.

Creativity is more than the making or the doing of something. Young (1985) explains that the word 'creativity' derives from the Latin 'creare' (to make) and the Greek 'Krainein' (to fulfil). He refers to the paradoxical nature of creativity as an integration of doing and being, and that the creator becomes something more through the act of creating. We have often witnessed the growth in people, in confidence and in presence, through creative process.

My passion for creative connections comes from my understanding of creativity as an energy that flows in all our lives. The more I work in this field, the more I regard creativity as the essence of life. It is thrilling that more people are recognising the positive and powerful effects of creativity on mental well-being and self-esteem. We seem to experience creativity as a *feeling*, as much as we see, hear or touch it. The doing and the being are integrated.

This too is our experience of puppetry. There is the act of creating the puppet, which might be from paper, fabric, wood or recycled objects. Then there is the animation of the puppet. Breathing life into something that was previously inanimate. The process of animation requires a particular way of being, which we can all learn. Sometimes, as can be seen in the book, the puppet appears to take on an 'aliveness', regardless of the skills of the puppeteer.

What you will find in this book

Following this introduction, Chapter 1 offers remarkable insights about the world of puppetry. We see why people with dementia respond so well. The work is not art therapy, but it does offer therapeutic value. Puppetry has a long association with restoration and well-being, from the African healing rituals and ceremonies, to puppets used by therapists with children traumatised by war or abuse. The chapter briefly describes the different forms of puppetry we use with adults living with dementia and refers to the puppet-making guides in the appendices. The term *applied puppetry* is used occasionally, as a reminder that the puppets are not being used to 'entertain' (although entertainment happens). Their primary purpose is as an application to a creative process for well-being.

The puppet stories in Chapter 2 convey the importance of understanding individual needs and life preferences. In the story of Helen and the kitten, her preference was strong and clear. Other people may prefer a variety of activities. It is quite possible (although rare in our experience) that someone might choose not to engage with puppetry at all. Each person's decision must be respected. There are still other ways to connect, other ways to care. Creativity has no boundaries.

The Department of Health and the World Health Organization promote the need to understand how individuals want to be cared for from their perspective. Being person-centred means finding out what matters to the individual. There is greater movement for people to be involved in decisions affecting their life and care plans. The chapter explores ways of discovering and honouring individual preferences through creativity. BICEPS is a set of principles using creativity and person-centred principles to connect with people whose voices have traditionally been unheard.

Chapter 3 is about responding to changes in relationship. The puppet stories show opposite ends of the spectrum that relatives and carers find themselves on. One story involves a carer who wants everything to be back to the way it was, with everyone in their roles, and all memory function restored. That need is palpable and poignant through all the creative activities we shared. The other story is of a carer who found new and rewarding ways to be with her relative. This shifting of roles in relationship is undoubtedly one of the areas carers find most difficult to achieve. But when they do, the way opens for connecting more deeply in other ways. The chapter uses the metaphor of a map to understand the journey the caregiver and care-receiver navigates to experience 'wonderment'.

These carer stories contain complex issues about our human desire to fix things, to make things better. Our cultural and personal values may feel challenged when someone behaves differently. Many people living with the late stages of dementia experience these challenges in their relationships. Through creativity we can discover new aspects of each other and ourselves.

Knowing how to communicate beyond words and memory is the subject of Chapter 4. Many of us are used to speaking, talking, chatting, gossiping, conversing, discussing. It can feel bewildering to be confronted with confused words, broken sentences or no words at all. In our uncertainty we tend to withdraw from the contact. And yet there are myriad ways to connect beyond spoken language.

Working with silence is a beautiful art that also benefits the caregiver. Students of my counselling courses thought they would find this the most difficult aspect to learn. Yet it often became a favourite request when they understood and felt the power of silent connection. This chapter's puppet stories show ways to work beyond the words. Not speaking allows us to be more aware of body language. You may already know the majority of our communication about personal or emotional matters happens through non-verbal language anyway. Having more confidence in connecting without words opens up a range of enjoyable encounters. We also work in silence with people who have visual impairment.

Chapter 5 is about connecting in times of conflict or confusion. People respond to their changing situations in different ways. Not knowing where you are or who anyone is can be extremely frightening, unless the person has a strong sense of being safe. Usual responses to fear are to withdraw or attack. One story gives an example of how puppets can step in and lift the person from their war zone.

Dealing with difficult situations is an area many carers ask for guidance on. It is important for each of us to feel safe in life. Conflict can be due to memory loss, or confused visual perceptions, which the carer must learn to negotiate.

My background includes working with people who communicated through anger and aggression. This behaviour is usually due to emotional turmoil or intense fear. But there are many triggers to be aware of. Sometimes the carer becomes the target of a rage against loss of independence, or other deep anguish. This chapter explains effective de-escalation techniques. Puppetry can help a person express their feelings, which is seen later on in the book. The underlying principle of this chapter is maintaining a focus on individual qualities and positive connections.

One way of preventing situations from escalating is to look at how a person's day is filled. Boredom is in itself a stressor. A meaningful life is the subject of Chapter 6. In discussions with staff or carers who work with people in the later stages of dementia, I ask: 'What makes a life worth living?' I am often struck by the immediate silence. It is as though we are all suspended in time and space, as we consider the meaning – I always find the answers inspiring.

In the past our society dismissed older people, and people with dementia. There was a collective sense that their lives were somehow less worthy. People justified these prejudices in terms of saying 'He's had a good life, it's someone else's turn now' or 'She's had enough. It will be a blessing when she pops her clogs.' The idea of therapeutic input for people with dementia was more or less rejected. Things have changed for the better.

Although concerns about ageist attitudes still exist, there is growing awareness of the need to value all people in our society. The chapter highlights the importance of increasing feelings of self-worth. The stories show two men helping to build puppets and a small theatre. Being involved in the creation of something for themselves and other people is stimulating and empowering. Having a sense of purpose, relevant to the individual, increases quality of life.

I often use a combination of applied puppetry with life story work or narrative work. Since 2003 we have made many memory boxes with people at home or in care settings, and you will find other ideas for enjoyable stimulation. In Chapter 7 I show how narrative work and puppetry can be done as a social group activity, with teamwork and conversation. Sometimes people are able to express how it feels to have dementia through their puppet. People may experience distress or fear about not being able to remember something. They may also find it very funny or awe-inspiring to be forced into the moment of 'Now' every day.

Themed days can also be wonderful experiences in care settings, as well as enjoyed in domestic homes. Some people enjoy having a restful, quiet life. Other people enjoy surprises and welcome opportunities to celebrate. There are many themes to be explored, some of which may involve a wider circle of people; other themes can be explored on a more personal basis.

Singing is widely known to have both physical and mental benefits for a wide range of people. It is so uplifting and of course we have singing puppets, which often add humour. Chapter 8 is dedicated to this energising activity. Research also shows how the singing helps people feel calm and connected. You may know that songs and music are often more easily retrieved than other memories. We have met many people who had stopped talking due to frustration over their loss of words, but who sing all the words to songs they knew. Organisations such as the Alzheimer's Society offer 'Singing for the Brain' sessions.

Chapter 9 brings us to the marvellous world of bed theatre. I have long been interested in how we ensure that our work is inclusive of people who, through illness, disease or disability, remain isolated in their beds. Sensitivity towards individual levels of engagement are always required. Bed-bound people often have long periods with little going on around them. It is important to build the activities a bit at a time, so as not to overwhelm anyone.

Sometimes, puppet work allows a connection to be made that would otherwise have been difficult to discover. One of the stories shows how the puppet work enabled staff to understand a situation differently and gain confidence in engaging with someone who was very frail. The activity can turn out to be the opposite of what we might expect. Puppets dare to do or say things that most of us wouldn't consider. They can bridge a gap – make the way for more human interaction and bring out individual personalities.

Having a sense of identity is important. There are many social and psychological theories about our individuality and identity. We might maintain self-identity through our values, our work, the groups we join, the things we do, or through the objects and people in our lives. When carers talk about dementia, this is an area that concerns them. Chapter 10 explores ways we use puppetry to highlight feelings of self, regardless of memories.

The stories are moving and yet uplifting as we see what is possible with people whose memories or words are being expressed differently. Validating individual experiences is an important part of the work.

For a long time reminiscence therapy was considered to be the answer to dealing with dementia. It certainly has an important role and is actively encouraged in many care settings. Many people enjoy discussing events of the past and recognising the richness of life. It is important these activities include non-verbal elements for people experiencing later stages of dementia. Chapter 11 looks at enjoyable and relaxing memory stimulation experiences, including old puppets. These activities suit people who struggle with the pressure of memory quizzes or are disadvantaged by the verbal exchanges often used in reminiscence work.

Many people have memories of pets. Animals can bring a special energy into the home. We've seen the great pleasure a big floppy-eared rabbit can bring to a hospice, or the love of cats who purr like outboard engines, and dogs who roll over for a belly rub. Pets can motivate people who are withdrawn, or calm people who are anxious. The mixture of stimulation and gentle appeal is probably why animal puppets are so well received. Chapter 12 shows examples of how glove puppet cats and dogs, and shop-bought soft-material animals can be used with dignity and respect for the person with dementia.

People's lives can be enhanced through small and simple acts of creativity and stimulation, just as much as through the bigger projects. Chapter 13 shows the value of even one tiny creative connection. It is important for staff and carers to get a sense of what they can easily achieve within a busy week, and to really know that this can make a positive difference. Staff and carers report feeling more motivated and inspired as a result. Caring can be draining, so it is important to find moments of joyfulness. This undoubtedly has a positive effect on the person being cared for.

Some carers may be in a position to support a few minutes of daily mental stimulation or learning therapy, as Kawashima (2012) calls it. His research with older people shows improved working memory and other thinking abilities. This is with people in all stages of dementia. There are more studies indicating the effectiveness of mental stimulation (or cognitive stimulation therapy – CST). We share a few ideas for incorporating creative mental stimulation and connection in daily life routines. These are things we can all be doing for ourselves starting now. It is in all our interests to be as physically fit and well as we can be.

The final two chapters look at puppetry as both passive and participative entertainment. Chapter 14 is about puppetry as entertainment for older people. There is a long tradition of puppet theatre, which can inspire exciting childhood memories. Some care homes are able to buy in professional entertainment. People enjoy watching the performers put everything together as much as they enjoy watching the show. However, this chapter is primarily for carers, activity coordinators or performers interested in entertaining in a domestic home or in a care home.

The chapter contains a sample script for puppet characters we have fun with. Often these performances work well without a set or scenery, but I have included instructions on how to make a simple booth for those who would prefer a set.

There is much fun to be had from do-it-yourself shows, involving older people who use care services or people living with dementia. Chapter 15 pulls together the various techniques described throughout the book for people to create their own performance art. The puppets, the sets, the sounds and scripts contain many aspects that can be broken down into user-friendly steps. We describe the process and highlight the importance of ensuring tasks are accessible, achievable, meaningful and above all else – enjoyable.

Ideas are given for intergenerational work as well as the power of using puppetry to convey messages to a wider public. The chapter explores the strengthening of community links for dementia friendly communities, and the role of people with dementia, carers and families to use creativity in that process.

Note

1.   Recorded phrases at the International Conference of Alzheimer's Disease held in London in March 2012.

CHAPTER 1

Old Joe Knows a Few Things

The World of Puppetry

Joe's door is open. He is spending time in bed following a fall. Mostly he tells visitors and staff to go away. He seems to think they are after his money. The puppeteers walk past his room and Joe notices two brightly coloured puppets dancing around.

'Hellooo,' he shouts, 'Come in, come in, come and visit old Joe.'

The two 'mouth puppets' are about the size of three-year-olds, each with a larger-than-life set of eyes and red mouth. Joe pats his bed, for them to sit beside him. The puppeteers settle on his bed, with the puppets facing Joe. Joe looks tired, but he stares at the big-eyed faces adoringly. The puppeteers remain still.

'Well,' he laughs, 'what have you got for old Joe today?'

He is speaking to the girl puppet. She stands on his bed and sings him a song and a nursery rhyme. Joe claps his hands and joins in with some of the words.

'You are so clever,' he tickles the puppet's stomach and she laughs.

'Now, young man,' he turns to the other puppet, 'can you beat your sister?'

The other puppet stands and recites the three times table, which Joe mouths along with him. The puppet falters after 3 x 6, but Joe keeps him right. They reach 3 x 15! After all this exertion, Joe asks the puppets for a kiss on his cheek. They give him a hug, which involves the puppeteers, puppets and Joe in a general bundle! As they are about to leave Joe looks at the puppeteers.

'Thank you, they seem so alive!' he says. Then he returns to waving to the puppets. 'Goodbye now my bairns, come and see old Joe another day.'

This ability for adults to fully enter the world of play, and yet be aware of the fact that they are responding to puppets is a regular occurrence. I enjoy this human capacity to move in and out of different realms. Beryl, a lady in her nineties, has been chatting to some more puppets and patting their heads.

'Oh my God!' exclaims her daughter, 'She thinks they're real. It's spooky!'

Without turning away from the puppets, Beryl whispers loudly to her daughter out of the corner of her mouth (as though she does not want the puppets to hear):

'I know what they are. I know they're puppets!'

Then she pats the puppets again, and talks to them as though they are indeed real. She laughs and sings to them; she stares at them intently and copies their movements. Not once does Beryl acknowledge the puppeteers, nor look at her daughter. This non-acknowledgement can be upsetting for relatives and carers. I explore this emotive and complex subject more fully in Chapter 3 about changes in relationships.

Beryl has a diagnosis of fronto-temporal lobe dementia, also referred to as FTD (for further information, see Alzeimher's Society 2012; Neary *et al.* 1990). This affects parts of the brain that deal with personality, reasoning, movement, speech, social skills, language and some aspects of memory. The deterioration of the front part of the brain may affect individual ability to empathise or show any concern for others. They may also lose their inhibitions in public, although some people withdraw from all social contact.

As with all diagnoses, there are variations in how individuals are affected. While Beryl seems unconcerned with staff and relatives, she readily engages with the puppets, and appears emotionally involved with them. It is during the following session that her daughter connects with Beryl in the world of puppetry.

Beryl is talking to the puppets. Some words are indiscernible, but it sounds light-hearted and caring. The daughter joins in by speaking to one of the puppets. Beryl stops momentarily and beams at her daughter, as though they are best buddies sharing something wonderful. And the feeling of connection is real, albeit fleeting. We all sense it. Beryl and her daughter relax together.

Beryl's memory is still intact, but her family notice her behaviour towards others has changed. Sometimes she may even seem uncaring in her dismissal of people. This could be due to the effects of the fronto-temporal lobe dementia. However, it is also clear that Beryl enjoys sharing imaginative recreation. Beryl's experiences remind us that individuals have their own rules and their own ways of coping with life and dementia.

Regular communication can be charged with all sorts of tensions that overwhelm a person living with dementia. The world of puppetry can be an enjoyable meeting space between people who, for whatever reason, have difficulty engaging in the ways we are used to.

There is something about creativity that releases people from the confines of a label. It does not mean that people are cured of disease, or miraculously change personalities. But there is a 'something else' that becomes visible, which may have been invisible before the creative encounter. This something else is what we call 'possibility'.

It is the possibility of connection. Puppets engage people in imaginary worlds, a world between worlds, open to anyone. Creativity and imagination have no boundaries, no exclusion zones. Puppets have a universal appeal. They connect with us on an emotional level. We are somehow wired to connect to the magical life breathed into inanimate objects. It is why puppetry is used in so many adverts on television.

In care work, puppetry creates a space, a meeting place, where verbal language, memory and questions do not have to be invited. Puppets have a visual and physical presence that attracts curiosity. They intrigue us. In that interesting, imaginative area we can share a positive and meaningful connection (see Figure 1).

People diagnosed with dementia or other long-term conditions affecting communication still have emotions, imagination, humour and sensitivities. Our work is to invite people to engage in creative connection, where these qualities are celebrated. Sometimes people need time to become aware of the offer to engage with us, and even longer to begin to participate. Other times the response is immediate. Either way, the connection builds. Creativity begets itself.

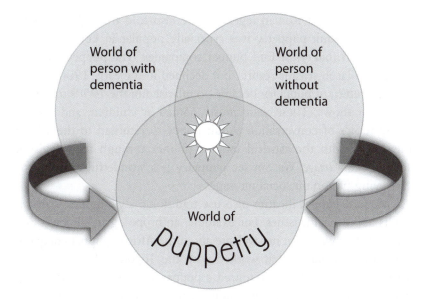

Figure 1 Puppet meeting space (Marshall 2008)

Puppetry for adults

I would like to clarify that puppets have a very adult history. This can help carers feel more comfortable with the concept of using this art form. It is thought the earliest puppets began in Asia for storytelling and sharing news and ideas about religion. We can imagine audiences around campfires watching shadow puppets made from animal hide.

In central West Mali, there is a long tradition of animal mask dances accompanied by little wooden people. These are used to represent ancestral stories and African legends, as well as an understanding of human psychology. Arnoldi (1995), an anthropologist, explains that each new generation is expected to create new characters to rival the old ways. The puppet and mask rituals help the society develop and move on.

> What is certain is that the puppet and the puppet play in different forms has existed since the earliest times, and [is] fundamental to the development of humankind. (Blundall 2012)

In the UK puppetry was used to pass social and political comment around towns and villages through country fair performances. Bible stories, Greek and Roman legends were also told through travelling puppeteers. Adult puppetry was especially popular in London in the 1700s, with four West End puppet companies. The puppets became more familiar in seaside resorts, but declined in the early 1900s.

The return of puppetry became popularised in the 1950s to 1970s television shows. These were mostly aimed at children, and can be useful topics of conversation. Adult puppetry returned to the UK in the 1980s with the satirical look at politics through the television show *Spitting Image*. We can see puppetry is a wonderful medium for conveying important social messages.

Modern puppet theatres also use traditional-style figures to teach adults about health issues. For example, anthropologist Elisabeth den Otter (1993) writes on her website about the African puppet company (Compagnie Danaye) that worked with the Togolese Association for Women against Aids. They toured a puppet show in 1993 educating people about Aids. I often use puppetry to explore issues about mental ill-health and recovery, and to raise public awareness.

Puppetry also has meaning beyond education and passing on information. The ancient practice of making human and animal figurines for rituals, rites and healing can be found throughout the world. These symbolic figures are often regarded as holding inner powers, and must be respected.

There is something awesome about sensing life in an item made of clay or wood or cloth. A puppet is more than an object, although objects can be puppets. Puppetry is the term used for bringing an object to life. To animate something is to breathe life into it. This takes a little practice, but creates magic and an emotional response in ways that do not always work between humans.

In West Africa, in Burkina Fasovast, around the Ivory Coast and Ghana, members of the Lobi tribe use wooden and clay figures called boteba. These are applied to a wide range of medical, healing and life event interventions.

Families request the boteba to commune with the invisible spirits of nature (thil) for protection and healing. Roy (2002) explains how they can additionally perform interim tasks such as finding lost items. The figures are also believed to have the power to communicate with each other independently. They act on behalf of their owners, and can bring harm or good fortune.

Beresford (1966) writes about Persian soldiers who took their favourite puppets to war with them for protection against the ancient Greeks. Many people carry good luck charms, and we see examples of this practice from corn dollies used to invoke wealth and success, to holy objects offering protection against evil spirits.

There are stories of wooden statue puppets being made by priests. Bussell (1968) explains how the priests would secretly move the limbs on the statues, so people thought they were witnessing God's power in the miracle of animation. This was supposedly done to strengthen people's faith.

Anyone who has experienced the enchantment of puppetry knows a sense of wonderment. We might laugh at ourselves for engaging with a puppet, yet we do it anyway. We connect emotionally to a piece of wood or cloth. We may even have a glimmer of speculation that 'something-other-than-my-world' exists. This feeling of wonder takes us into the realm of possibility. Our minds open.

From wonder into wonder, existence opens. (Laozi 1989, p.31)

Agatha is in her late nineties. She seems to sleep most of the time and waves her carers away when they offer her drinks. Staff are concerned that Agatha is becoming seriously dehydrated. They try music, hand massages and magazines for stimulation. She shuts her eyes. When she opens them, Agatha sees a puppet at her door. She looks surprised; her eyes light up and she whispers as she smiles.

'Oh, look at that! Look at that!'

Agatha beckons the puppet over. We settle at the end of her bed. The puppet gives a mini-performance. Agatha beams. Gradually, we are invited to look at photographs of her family. The carer sits with Agatha, helping her drink through a straw, while Agatha's eyes are fixed on the puppets moving things around her bed. She is clearly in the world of peaceful delight.

The secret of this art [puppetry] is to be found in the magic when an inanimate object creates an emotional contact with a human spectator. May this magic never die. (Speaight 1990, p.359)

Using puppets with people with dementia

Over the years of working in care and community settings, I have noticed that applied puppetry and creativity positively affect people's emotional states. We all benefit in some way from creativity. As passive recipients we appreciate the music that soothes us, the comedian who makes us laugh, the drama that moves us, the aesthetic power of art that lifts our mood.

An in-depth review by Staricoff (2004) of 385 research studies and medical literature shows a wealth of evidence about the positive impact of arts for reducing medication, reducing stress levels and increasing cognitive function. For example people with dementia are reported to have better memory function and word recall following music, singing or other creative arts session.

This rise in awareness and ability is often reported in our work. Carers at home say their relatives become more talkative after the puppet session. One man said he felt his brain was oiled with the laughter and enjoyment.

Clearly stimulation is important, as will be seen throughout this book. Having something interesting to consider or participate in helps raise pleasure levels, which increases self-esteem. When motivation strikes us, it seems as though our capabilities expand. We gain confidence and feel more energised, which stimulates more parts of the brain. Cognitive stimulation therapy is valuable in dementia care, and is discussed further in Chapter 13.

The majority of my work is about connecting with people who desire to be connected. I facilitate communication to express experiences, feelings and desires through the medium of puppetry. Helping people create their own puppet is deeply rewarding. We may see the puppet become an extension of the individual. It communicates or interacts with other puppets or people, often with great humour and insight.

For example, two older ladies began communicating with each other through their puppets. They shared the same care home, but had not conversed before. Many people living in the home seemed self-contained. Not being disturbed by anyone has its merits for those of us who enjoy solitude. But through the puppets we discovered that people wanted to be in connection with other people. They had been nervous about approaching each other.

One lady did not use verbal language, but through her puppet, she engaged with the other lady. They spent a merry afternoon puppeteering their cartoon style versions of themselves on a small stage. There was interaction between the puppets, and much laughter. On another day, the two ladies sat beside each other and painted a backcloth for the theatre. They developed camaraderie.

In his work about social issues around the world, puppeteer Gary Friedman (2010) talks about the power of puppetry to enable people to express themselves and break down any barriers that might exist. We consistently see this magic at work. From managers of big organisations to the frail lady tucked up in her bed, people speak to puppets. They cross any boundaries and create a level playing field.

> [We see] a symbolic self-representation that is three-dimensional; it is a communicative modality that speaks, interacts, and 'lives' in a way that much two-dimensional art does not. (Holloway 2011)

Janie's wooden puppet wore tinted glasses (made from coloured cellophane) just like hers. She concentrated hard to move her hand, which was the only part of her body with mobility, as she painstakingly painted the wooden puppet body. Janie chose hair that matched her own.

When asked if her puppet also needed a wheelchair, Janie nodded. But she changed her mind. She pointed to bright material for the clothes and moved the puppet in the air. Soon the puppet in its yellow and blue dress danced freely. Janie whispered 'dancing queen'.

Puppets can do things that people can't. Janie's carers were able to build on the dancing theme because Janie showed them what she liked through her puppet.

So, we see that puppetry works with different people and on different levels:

- Puppets tell stories or pass on information.

- Puppets are imbued with powers of healing, wonderment or spirituality.

- Puppetry is an activity for passive or participative enjoyment.

- Puppetry is for self-expression and of therapeutic value.

Each of these ways has relevance for working with people with dementia, whether at home, in a day centre or in a care home. The puppet work can be as complex or easy as desired, and is suitable for all stages of dementia including late stages and end of life care.

Puppets connect with people in ways that do not rely on words or memory, so we have found them highly effective. They are non-threatening. In a world where everyone may appear to be a stranger and places seem unfamiliar, it is still possible to find enjoyment and laughter. We connect in the moment of 'now'.

The puppet can present exaggerated aspects of individuals, and generate genuine feelings of pride, love, sadness and joyfulness. People sometimes find it easier to initially express themselves through creativity, than through face-to-face human contact. The human connection is still present, but in a less obvious way. Puppets are one step removed from the intensity of daily life and expectations. Serious issues can be explored with humour, with or without words.

The appendices show puppet-making ideas so you can get started on an activity. But first it is worth considering which type of puppet might best suit you or the person or people you are with.

Different forms of puppetry

It is helpful to understand what suits various physical and cognitive capacities. It is important to ensure the task is accessible, achievable and appropriate.

For example, if Mr Brown has painful arthritis in his hand, we will work with a lightweight puppet that is easy to manoeuvre. If Mrs MacInnes is unable to control excessive saliva or drooling, we use materials that can be washed. Working in well-lit rooms is very important as the eyesight of older people may deteriorate, and half-lit rooms appear very dark. The importance of being person-centred and adapting to individual needs is shown in Chapter 2 and throughout the book.

The following overview shows some of the puppets that can be used for stand-alone activity sessions, as well as for a process of connection over several months. All of these appear in various stories highlighted through the book.

Model theatre puppets are based on the paper puppetry from 200 years ago. There is simplicity about making paper or cardboard representations of people, which can be done individually or in groups. We find people generally love this activity, especially the cartoon-style puppets.

Marionettes are string puppets, usually with movable limbs, head, shoulders and body. They are probably one of the most complex puppet forms to make and puppeteer using two hands, but they are highly appreciated. For people who enjoy problem solving, challenges and longer-term projects, this is the puppet for you! We help people make marionette versions of themselves, and a simpler marionette bird.

Tabletop puppets also have jointed moving parts, but are held by a rod in the back of the head or body, instead of strings. We find these puppets (which measure 20–30cm) are very desirable, as they can be used with one hand. The making of them can be broken down into stages. There is a degree of dexterity required, but with help all sorts of things can be achieved.

Pom-pom puppet-making is a social activity. In one care home, we had pom-poms being made by the people living in the home, nurses, relatives, the social worker, the handy-man and the health visitor! They can be made easily at home too. There is an olde-worlde comforting feel to the task, although the knot-tying bit at the end may require supple fingers. The pom-pom woollen balls can be strung together using a thick needle and thread, or simply sit on glued felt feet, with glued-on eyes.

Mouth puppets have a big presence. We make our own, but it is much easier to use or adapt ready-made ones. The hand is placed inside the head to make the mouth open and close. People who have impaired vision often enjoy these puppets with their big mouths and large eyes. They are ideal as singing puppets.

Vintage puppets are the ones many people would be familiar with from their childhood. We use Lambchop and Pinky and Perky puppets along with some of the 1950s Pelham Puppets. Images of them can be useful too for conversations and trips down memory lane.

Animal puppets, especially cats and dogs, bring great pleasure. We use the animals in bed-theatre work as well as for conversation topics, and for silent comedy work.

Shadow puppets can be terrific for group work and for creating immediate puppet shows. The making of the puppets is easily attainable. It can also be highly artistic, depending on the needs of people involved. However, the task involves switching lights on and off, as the shadow puppets are projected onto a bright screen in the darkness. We find that people in mid to late stages of dementia need more time for their eyes to adjust to the lighting levels.

Glove puppets (hand puppets) are one of my favourites, because they are so alive. People enjoy creating versions of themselves as they are today, but we have also worked with people creating representations of themselves in a previous role or occupation. The puppets are usually sewn. We sometimes prepare the basic glove puppet for the person to dress and decorate.

Sock puppets are great for puppet-making novices. When activities are new to a person, having a task that can be attained within a few minutes helps to boost confidence. When concentration or memory is short, the sock puppet making session is perfect. We also use them for participative and humorous singing sessions. Sock puppets seem instantly comical.

Object puppetry requires a belief in the objects' ability to be alive. We use scarves, cutlery, lampshades, shirts – anything that may resonate with the person. There is usually nothing to make. The object is moved in such a way as to express an emotion or become something else. Object puppetry allows imagination and innovation to flourish.

While on the subject of objects, I would like to mention ephemeral puppetry, or *ephemeral animation*, a term created by Watson (2011) to describe objects that move without human control. Their movement is created by natural elements such as wind or water. Sometimes we pay attention to these movements.

I remember sitting at the bedside of a lovely lady in her late nineties, as she lay dying. I had been her nurse for a few months, and we had shared many hours of reading and chatting. Her family needed a break from their constant vigil. As I listened to her tiny breaths, I held her hand and gazed out of the window.

Earlier I had washed one of her long nightdresses and hung it from the hem on the washing line, and I could see it gently flapping around. Suddenly the nightdress was swept up with the wind. It caught in the birch tree, as though standing on the washing line. This lively tightrope walker mesmerised me. I told the lady what her nightdress was doing. She opened her eyes and smiled. Then she fell into a deep sleep and I gathered her family to hold hands with her as she passed away. It was a very peaceful, gentle death.

Ephemeral puppetry does not have to have any rhyme or reason to it. A set of circumstances come together and something moves in an unexpected way that catches our attention. We are in the moment. For me, puppetry, with or without a puppeteer, has a Zen-like quality. For others, the flapping of a plastic bag on a fence is just a plastic bag on a fence, but try noticing these moments. You will be seeing puppetry everywhere!

CHAPTER 2

Kissing Scarves

Being Person-Centred

Mrs P. sits up straight on the chair facing the front door of the care home. She comes in for respite care and spends the majority of the time awaiting the arrival of her daughter to take her home. Mrs P. wears a beautiful tweed skirt and jacket, with a pale pink blouse and flowery silk scarf around her neck. One delicate hand checks her hair is all in place, the other holds tight to the strap of her small leather bag on her lap.

When Mrs P. is invited to participate in activities, she politely declines. Her immaculate clothes and self-containment exemplify dignity. She appears not to need anything. It is noticeable after a week that staff have stopped making suggestions or inviting Mrs P. to participate. She glances only fleetingly when we arrive and shows no interest in any of the puppets. She remains straight, but her fingers are restless. Her fingers tap her bag and chair. She pats at her beautiful scarf, tucking the ends inside her jacket.

At the next session, I wear a silk scarf and sit near Mrs P. and remove my scarf to shake it out. Mrs P. looks over. I take another scarf from my pocket and shake that one out too. But when I look at Mrs P., she looks away. I refocus on the scarves. By tying three knots in the first scarf I create a simple puppet with a head and hands. The puppet begins as a crumpled heap and grows into a tall, confident character exploring its surroundings. Mrs P. watches and smiles. I offer the second scarf to her and together we create another puppet.

Mrs P. moves her puppet by mirroring my actions, making the scarf puppet stretch its hand and lift its head, to rise in the air. My puppet stands on the arm of the chair and looks around and points at things. The second puppet looks and copies. I hum a waltz 'The Blue Danube' for the puppets to dance to. We are in connection. After a few minutes, Mrs P. makes her puppet touch noses with my puppet, as though giving a kiss. She speaks for the first time in our encounter:

'I think they like each other.'

Prior to this connection, the staff had made statements about Mrs P. based on their experiences of her:

'She wants to be left alone.'

'She does not like other people.'

Neither of these statements was entirely correct. The staff believed they were being sensitive to Mrs P.'s needs and preferences, based on their observations. They stopped inviting Mrs P. to join in activities, because she always declined. They felt the care was honouring Mrs P. and was therefore person-centred. But the focus was on their interpretations of Mrs P., and not on the lady herself. We are all capable of making such assumptions. We may know someone for years or for a few minutes, and if we rely on rational assessments, without 'tuning in', we may be far from the truth.

Assumptions may be partially true, or true for a particular time or not true at all. If we all continue responding to our own statements, the focus of our care is not on the person. This is a common problem that can lead to a narrowing of choices and reduce the prospects for relationship building. Another danger of maintaining an assumption about a person is that we limit opportunities for the person to respond differently.

Individual preferences and needs change depending on factors such as his or her level of confidence, well-being or pain. The environment and attitudes of the carer can also significantly affect the level of engagement. If opportunities are not there, or the environment does not resonate with them, people may experience increased isolation and poor mental health.

Being sensitive to individual needs requires us to consider the concept of individual resonance. What is of significance to the person? We need to find 'connection'. This is fundamental to meaningful communication.

We can see that Mrs P.'s appearance is important to her. However, what she wears is in contrast to other people in the home. The staff have plain uniforms and comfortable shoes. Some carers have their hair tied back but many do not appear to have had time to do much with their appearance. Our own clothes are just as casual. People living in the care home are in various states of dress: baggy trousers on the gentleman who is losing weight; fallen stockings bunching around the ankles of a lady; saliva stains on the shirt of another gentleman.

There is discord between Mrs P.'s values and what is present in the home. From the world of dignified, beautiful clothes there is nothing to relate to, not even a picture on the wall to reflect her preferences. When a person has nothing to relate to, he or she becomes increasingly self-contained and sometimes fearful. In such a situation it is likely that all further invitations to participate are declined, because without a sense of connection, nothing can develop.

It was not the puppet that Mrs P. responded to, for she was not initially interested in any of the other puppets. It was the acknowledgement of what is important to her. Beautiful clothes, dignity, the silk scarf. On its own the silk scarf did not generate the relationship, but there was a connection. The puppetry allowed this connection to build without words, in a way that Mrs P. could express herself, and communicate the friendship. The words were the last part in this process.

We see that the first connection opens possibilities for more. We are more effective when we tune in and focus on the person as they truly are, rather than on our assumptions about them. Being person-centred in the care home or in the family home means understanding and responding to personal values, personal needs and experiences. In theory, person-centred care is easier to deliver in the domestic home. The care can be more flexible; the pattern and pace of the day more individual.

Person-centred care is a way of thinking about, and responding to, the person. A care organisation should uphold the following points:

- The service needs to be right, from the perspective of the person for whom the service is for.

- The person for whom the service is for, is the expert on what suits and does not suit him or her.

This is further captured in the UK Department of Health (DOH) reports on personalisation:

every person who receives support, whether provided by statutory services or funded by themselves, will be empowered to shape their own lives and the services they receive in all care settings. (DOH 2008)

Person-centred care is highlighted as *essential* for quality care. Focus on the person is promoted by the World Health Organization (2010) placing people-centred care at the heart of primary care around the world. The 'Geneva Declaration on person-centred care for chronic diseases' (*International Journal of Person-centred Medicine* 2012) states that the twenty-first century is emerging as 'the century of person-centred care'. Dementia care strategies all emphasise person-centred approaches (see e.g. Scottish Government 2011).

What stops people being person-centred?

Part of the issue, also noticed by Brooker (2004), is that the term 'person-centred care' sounds wonderful but people do not know how to put it into practice. Some carers even doubt it is possible for everyone. This chapter looks at some of the historical and current issues and gives examples of when care is and is not person-centred.

Carers recognise that well-being is holistic; they aim to meet physical, emotional, social, mental and spiritual needs. This is a marked improvement from the long-established care services. Policies and procedures in the past were mainly concerned with just the physical aspects of care (the disease or the disability). Other needs were less catered for, although staff did their best within these structures.

The requirements of the organisation were paramount over the needs of the individual. Care services had (and still do need) to be financially viable, efficient and sustainable. However, when this means the service limits personal choices and does not recognise individual needs, we have 'institutionalisation'. This can occur in any setting, as it is established in attitudes and systems. The culture of an organisation (or a family) determines how institutionalised the setting is.

Goffman (1961) described the effects of institutionalisation. When the system limits choices and restricts quality experiences, there is depression and lack of spontaneity. These processes are in evidence in some group homes, especially where communication and interactions are poor, or where the culture is not open to feedback. The person is not at the centre of the service. The challenge for all of us is to minimise those processes.

Damaging effects happen more easily where there is great strain and stress. Individuals (staff, service users or relatives) may not recognise rights and choices for themselves or for each other. They may not be able to see beyond the challenges they face. However, there is progress. At least people have heard of person-centred care! There is worldwide acknowledgement that individuals are valuable.

Cost is often declared a major barrier to extending or adapting services. But not all things cost more, and the cost of not changing may be greater. Paid or unpaid carer burnout and stress have high physical and emotional costs, which all translate into financial costs (for the health system, employment sector and tax payer).

The need to increase awareness

Standards of care depend on our values, rules, knowledge, skills, awareness and understanding. Carers do what they learn how to do. This is influenced by their experiences; by how they were treated; their culture; learning; clarity of responsibilities; and their mental health. Carers may believe they are person-centred when they say:

> 'My day revolves around my wife, and it is tiring, so she goes to bed early to give me a break.'

> 'Our clients get a choice of activities and meals.'

> 'We know what suits Eric and we always abide by that.'

But the above statements are flawed if, for example, the individual prefers to stay up late, or the choice of activity is between two things that do not appeal, or the assumption about Eric is not right. What makes a service person-centred is greater than the statements we make. Our values and beliefs influence how person-centred we are.

Carers might struggle to know how to care for someone in later stages of dementia, when there may be loss of speech, increased frailty, cognitive decline and loss of mobility. Lack of skills can lead to a person becoming more isolated and possibly neglected. We need creative ways to understand people whose language or cognitive ability is changed.

Mr Davis's carer does not know how to manage the risk of him falling, so she tips his chair back to such an angle that he cannot get out. Mr Davis's legs make rapid cycling movements in the air, like a beetle flaying around on its back. He alternately cries in anguish and sleeps. With support, the carer learns less restrictive and less distressing ways to care for Mr Davis.

Going back over his life history reveals that Mr Davis was a postman. Walking was a big part of his life. A handrail is fitted along the hallway. Mr Davis decides to walk sideways, holding the rail with both hands. Corners of furniture are padded. He wears slippers that fasten properly to his feet.

Family members and neighbours are encouraged to write postcards or notes and drop them in the letter cage attached to the door. Mr Davis collects the mail from the door box, and puts it in his shoulder bag, to take back to the dining-room table. He is no longer distressed. He hums tunes to himself. There are more ways to connect with him.

The carer realised she had forgotten how to value Mr Davis. This can happen when the carer feels overwhelmed with the responsibility. Sometimes people need help to reflect on what is happening. Environments that offer regular supervision, or support, can help generate achievable person-centred ideas through mentoring and learning programmes.

Burnout or carer fatigue is a big sign to take notice of. Emotional, physical and mental exhaustion is caused by long periods of stress. This affects people in different ways, but gets in the way of person-centred care. Some people may be present in body, but emotionally shut down and seem to lose the ability to connect on a humane level.

Other people become hypersensitive to the suffering they see around them. They feel helpless and are in constant emotional pain. Either way requires intervention, support and change.

Many people go in to care work with good intentions. Family members care out of love and duty. The core care values resonate deeply with each of us. We all understand the human needs for dignity, respect, rights and choices, effective communication, self-worth, inclusion, privacy and protection from harm.

Some carers discover these purported values are not easily delivered within the care systems. When staffing levels are short or a regimented routine is in place, the staff do their best to keep delivering from the core values. But something happens to people, when the values that mean so much to them, are constantly hindered by the working environment or culture.

There is an internal conflict. The gap between what they want to do, and what they feel they actually can do, becomes increasingly difficult to deal with. It is at this point of stress that things happen. Staff might decide to leave and find a place that walks its talk, where they can deliver the good practice they believe in. Or they may become ill and go off sick, or become emotionally distant. Or they become increasingly frustrated and angry, possibly turning into bullies. These are all signs of burnout.

Family carers find it harder to walk away, but they still have these feelings to deal with. Family carers are more likely to suffer emotional or stress-related illnesses as a direct result of looking after someone (*British Medical Journal* 2007). Team leaders, family supporters and colleagues need to listen to carers who may be struggling. Person-centredness is not just for service users.

> Healthcare teams, healthcare provider organisations and governments often articulate an intention to deliver person-centred care. However, achieving it is often challenging and difficult to sustain. Achieving person-centred care consistently requires specific knowledge, skills and ways of working, a shared philosophy that is practiced by the nursing team, an effective workplace culture and organisational support. (Manley, Hills and Marriot 2011, p.35)

The values of person-centredness apply to everyone. It is useful to understand it in terms of the main elements found by Brooker. Her VIPS acronym is perfect for remembering the four elements:

- A *Value* base that asserts the absolute value of all human lives regardless of age or cognitive ability.

- An *Individualised* approach that recognises uniqueness.

- Understanding the world from the *Perspective* of the service user.

- Providing a *Social* environment that supports psychological needs.

(Brooker 2006, p.13)

Opportunities to gain person-centred care skills are essential. People can learn to fully appreciate the perspective of individuals whose language or life experience is changing. Each of us has a very personal understanding of life experience. In some aspects of life our knowledge and appreciation is very wide. In others, it is limited.

We might have a strong sense of how it feels to be unwell, or confined to bed. But we may not fully know what a person experiences when they are unable to make themselves understood. Our viewpoints may be limited. If we are aware of this, we can stay open to the fact that we may not be seeing all there is to see. The problem is that we do not know what we do not know, that is, we may not realise our view is limited (although we may sometimes sense there is something more!).

As people require more care and support, there is a tendency for staff and carers to do things from their perspective. They take control of all aspects of a person's life choices, treatment and direction. In their efforts to be caring, people sometimes fall into the trap of making assumptions. Carers fit people into their own ideas about what constitutes good care.

Eric sleeps in an armchair in the living room after lunch. When woken he is often upset and disorientated. Sometimes he seems rude or angry. The carers suggest it is better for his health and well-being if he is left to relax peacefully for the afternoon. They are very clear that Eric will not participate in the puppetry programme.

There is a logic and kindness to these statements. Staff have experiences of caring for many people and they often know what helps and doesn't help a person feel well. The danger, as I have seen in many care settings, is that the assumption about a person becomes a fact told in a different way. In this case the sentence is 'Eric is to miss every afternoon opportunity for enjoyment, connection, participation and communication.'

The carers draw these conclusions from their experiences of being shouted at and seeing the distress and upset on Eric's face when he is woken. They are caring for Eric, and they are doing their best for him, but they are also limiting his options.

Institutionalised thinking happens when we are not self-aware. It happens when we do not have time to reflect on the way we are working or thinking. Institutional ageism or dementia-ism (a term credited to Brooker 2004) is something to be alert to. This occurs, in the way institutional racism was found to exist, when the discrimination against an individual is inherent in the systems, policies and procedures. It is not necessarily the action of one individual against another, but a persistent way of thinking about individuals seen as belonging to a particular group or label.

When given the opportunity, staff connect with Eric quite quickly. He becomes one of the most active participants on the puppetry programme. He makes puppets and performs with them. He expresses his feelings and thoughts about dementia and inspires an atmosphere of enjoyment around him. His social experiences increase. He is more confident, less defensive.

The shift happens because people allow themselves to be open to the sense of possibility. They recognise the accidental discrimination that has taken place and change their attitudes. In this atmosphere of awareness, Eric, despite the confusion in his head, is able to shine.

Finding out about the person

When we know what a person likes or does not like, we can find ways to adapt the activities or interactions to be accessible. The knowledge that Mr Davis enjoyed post office work is adapted to suit his current situation. The following are ways in which we can discover what matters to an individual. Understanding individual values, likes, dislikes, strengths and needs helps to provide better care. If communication is difficult or cognitive function has changed, there are still ways to tune in and connect.

Verbal life history

This activity can be done at any time, with or without a diagnosis of dementia. More in-depth story work is shown in Chapter 10. A life history is often taken upon admission to a care setting, to help staff plan care. Family carers also find this a useful document to create for respite carers. The following aspects are usually covered, but you could add or subtract items depending on what seems appropriate:

- date of birth
- place of birth
- mother's and father's names and occupations
- childhood – where brought up/siblings/significant people/ games/school/achievements or events
- adulthood – big events/occupations/love/holidays/achievements
- home – layout/garden/partner/children/pets

- favourite things – hobbies/music/books/films/newspapers/food

- preferred things – times for getting up or going to bed/shower or bath

- spirituality – religion/place of worship/other information

- date the history was recorded or amended.

In middle and later stages of dementia, people may experience different time frames, or retrieve memories from the past more regularly. This life history can be useful for carers to understand and acknowledge what was important around that time.

The life story work may have less meaning in later stages, when people experience more 'in the moment' connections. However, reading someone's life story helps carers and visitors respect the humanity, social history, individuality and integrity of each person. This affirms the individual's personhood.

Generations of people through civil wars, slavery abolishing, other human rights issues and spirituality have considered the components of personhood. What makes us a person with rights? Kitwood (1997a) is recognised for extensive, compassionate and innovative development about person-centred care of people with dementia. His definition of personhood – 'a position or social relationship that is bestowed on one human being by "others" in the context of relationship and social being' – continues to be discussed.

At the heart of person-centred care is the person. When people take time to understand an individual, and plan the care with this knowledge in mind, quality of life is improved. Kitwood (1997a) is clear that an individual's well-being and quality of life are influenced by their history, their sensory awareness (eyesight, hearing and so on), their social and physical environments, their neurological impairment and their mental and physical health.

Observation

If the carer does not understand a person's cognition or language differences, observation of the person can help clarify what the person prefers in life. This is something I used to ask staff to do in the 1980s, when working with people with complex and multiple learning disabilities. Carers would take turns to observe, which encouraged self-reflective practice. Carers discussed what they noticed, such as:

- What attracts a person's attention and for how long?

- Who does the person enjoy seeing/being with?

- What does he or she enjoy doing?

- When does the person use vocal sounds most/least?

- What can the person do or not do for him or herself?

- Under what circumstances does the person withdraw or engage?

- What times of day is he or she most alert or tired?

Kitwood (1997b) developed a more formal observation tool in the 1990s, which is still used around the world. Known as Dementia Care Mapping (DCM), independent and trained 'mappers' observe interactions and behaviours over six-hour periods. Mappers generally work in pairs. They use codes to record various factors about the way a person behaves in the environment every five minutes. Factors that contribute to the person's well-being or lack of well-being are noted. The information is fed back to the staff. Again, this helps carers understand how to provide person-centred care.

Whether you do this formally or informally, scientifically or intuitively, it offers an important opportunity to sit back and consider what life is like from the perspective of the individual receiving care. Carers often notice factors in the environment they can improve, such as the temperature, lighting and noise levels, or the appropriateness of radio or TV programmes. Other things could be improvement in the directions given by staff, the length of time needed for a response, the best time of day to interact with the person.

Person-centred creative thinking

The physical environment and resources may influence person-centred care. Use creative thinking to get around obstacles.

Visits to or from service users in the community may be restricted due to staff work patterns or rural distances. But the use of digital technology and social media means some services can extend their reach. There are many online support forums, reaching people previously unable to get to sources of help.

Not everyone in a care home wants to have dinner with 30 people in a huge dining room. Some care homes are now creating more intimate dining spaces, by dividing the big room using partition walls. Walls at chest height also create multiple leaning surfaces. People who are unsteady on their feet find it much easier to move across a space in stages. Having something to hold onto a short distance away is reassuring.

Interestingly Johnson and Slater (1993) studied two comparable care homes, each with 42 people including individuals described as 'elderly confused'. The buildings were similar in style and layout. One care home continued functioning with the large communal dining area. A great amount of time was taken in helping people to and from this space, which was some distance from people's bedrooms. There was a high level of stress around the mealtimes, which I have also noticed in many care homes. Staff try to get everyone there on time, at least twice a day. Then there is the business of helping people to the toilet afterwards.

The other care home looked at their space differently. They found ways to create facilities closer to people's bedrooms, by turning the old sluice rooms at either end of the building into kitchenettes. They found spaces around the home to put tables, so people dined in groups of four or five, closer to their rooms. There were more handrails, which gave people added security and independence. People living at the home became more involved in serving themselves breakfast from the kitchenettes. Someone from each group collected the main meals on a trolley. Pushing a trolley was quite different from using a walking frame, because there was more of a sense of purpose about it.

This creative change in the care home had a huge impact. People became more self-sufficient, and helped one another in their small groups. There was a more respectful atmosphere, which included referring to people as Mr, Miss or Mrs as preferred. The level of one-to-one communication and interaction between staff and care-receivers significantly increased. Less time was spent on 'doing for' people, compared to the care home that stayed the same.

In short, the creative thinking of staff led to a more person-centred and fulfilling care service. This way of working also required fewer staff than the traditional care home. We have only just begun to realise the changes that care organisations can make. I find the conversations with design students so exciting, because they have such fresh vision for influencing care home cultures and improving quality of life in care settings.

To be person-centred we must be willing to question our own practice, values and rules. How wonderful if we all operated from person-centred values, beyond the statements:

> An effective workplace culture has a common vision through which values are implemented in practice and experienced by patients, service users and staff. (Manley *et al.* 2011, p.36)

Relationship-centred

One manager described how care staff found a deeper understanding of individual care needs following a puppetry programme. Over several weeks, people created puppets of themselves. They performed pieces about how they came to the care service. The puppets also highlighted what was personally important, or described a hope for each person. Staff had worked with many of the service users over several years. The expression through puppetry enabled staff members to see individual needs in a different way. Their relationships deepened and needs could be met more fully.

Appreciation of human individuality and motivation (Chapter 6) improves quality care, and promotes equality and diversity. Creativity offers an equitable framework to build caring relationships, which underpin care work. The creative interactions offer equal ground for expression, appreciation, connection, inclusion, communication, belonging, valuing, compassion, empowerment and enjoyment.

The term 'relationship-centred care' is sometimes used in addition to (or instead of) person-centred care. Nolan *et al.* (2004) suggest that the relationship approach to care is more appropriate for working with older people or people with dementia. He highlights the importance of belonging, feeling safe in the relationship, consistency, having goals and feeling valued.

Relationship-centred care considers the balance between independence, dependence and interdependence, rather than the person-centred individualistic emphasis. The negotiation of dependency is at the heart of many caregiver and care-receiver relationships. People try to hang on to their independence, fearful of becoming dependent. Interdependence means a reciprocal relationship, where both parties experience a sense of growth or benefit from being in relationship.

One carer I met said caring for her husband teaches her to take time to appreciate nature, and feel calmer about life, as they tend plants together. A paid member of staff finds great solace in giving care to people the same age as her parents, because she is on the other side of the world to her own family. There are numerous ways in which relationships can be reciprocal. Relationship-centred care can be regarded as a process of discovery.

> Contact with dementia or other forms of severe cognitive disability can – and indeed should – take us out of our customary patterns of over-busyness, hyper-cognitivism and extreme talkativity, into a way of being in which emotion and feeling are given a much larger place. People who have dementia, for whom the life of the emotions is often intense, and without the ordinary forms of inhibition may have something important to teach the rest of humankind [to return] closer to the life of instinct. (Kitwood 1997a, p.5)

Carers who find this way of being enjoy it! Artists and people who meditate may be more familiar with a state of beingness, but we probably all have experiences of it, particularly when something fills us with awe.

> Its essence silently communicates itself to you and reflects your own essence back to you. This is what great artists sense and succeed in conveying in their art. Van Gogh didn't say: 'That's just an old chair.' He looked, and looked, and looked. He sensed the Beingness of the chair. Then he sat in front of the canvas and took up the brush. The chair itself would have sold for the equivalent of a few dollars. The painting of that same chair today would fetch in excess of $25 million. (Tolle 2009, p.20)

Not every carer feels a sense of awe. Not every carer can get that sense of value when he or she feels overwhelmed. Family carers in particular may be dealing with huge challenges, distressing behaviour, aggression and self-harm, on top of feeling exhausted. Sometimes the best a carer can do is sit on the bed and cry. It may not sound very much like person-centred care. It probably is not awesome either. But if crying is the best that can be done on this day, then that is the best. Tomorrow is another day.

BICEPS

The process for connecting through creativity and joy involves the strength of BICEPS:

- *Breathing* into the moment.
- *Intention* to make the day as comfortable and as joyful as possible.
- *Creative* thinking.
- *Expectation* of connection, beyond personal or relationship constraints.
- *Practice* of person-centred counselling principles.
- *Self-awareness*.

Breathing

Applied puppetry works because life is breathed into the moment. This is explored further in Chapter 4.

Intention

There can be no better intention than making the day comfortable and joyful, although it will vary day to day.

Creative thinking

Already we have seen how creative thinking can change an environment, and there are more examples to follow.

Expectation

In the early stages of dementia, when memory and cognitive function are not so noticeable, carers expect to be recognised and remembered. Over the years, there may be less recognition. But I want to show how the expectation of connection can go beyond being personally recognised. It is about connecting in the moment of now – in a place that feels joyful and comfortable. In some ways it does not matter who does that connecting, so long as it is done with love. This subject is explored more in Chapter 3, because to reach that point requires a change in the relationship.

Person-centred counselling principles and self-awareness

The principles used in this work require practice and self-awareness. People tend to realise things in layers from intellectual understanding to the core of knowing, so I show these elements in different ways through the chapters.

Basic person-centred counselling begins with the belief that each person is an expert on himself or herself and knows what is best for their well-being. When working with people with profound and multiple disabilities, or conditions such as dementia, some carers throw up their hands like Andy Pandy (the puppet) at this idea. However, as James McKillop of the Scottish Dementia Working Group says:

> I believe that [people with dementia] can make a choice, be it an oral answer, a nod or shake of the head, or perhaps moving a part of their body such as a finger. The trick is to get to know how they best communicate and go down that line. (McKillop and Petrini 2011, p.333)

Rogers (2003) pioneered client-centred therapy (from which person-centred care in dementia care has developed) during the great period of human rights developments in the 1950s. Rogers believed that individuals have a natural motivating force for positive growth, and that we should not assume we know best about the life of another individual.

The understanding is that each person has within them the resources, gifts, wisdom, strength and power for emotional well-being. In order to support the individual, the carer or counsellor needs to demonstrate the following:

- *Unconditional positive regard* is a total respect for the person and acceptance of what is of value to the person. This helps the person feel valued.

- *Congruence* is genuine and appropriate behaviour that does not hide behind a professional role of facade. There is openness so the words are sincere. The carer's actions match what he or she says, thinks and feels. This helps the person feel safe.

- *Empathy* is the ability to enter the world of another person (as far as is possible), to understand how she or he perceives life, and then communicate this understanding. Being able to 'feel' with someone else, while remaining separate, helps the person feel understood.

(Rogers 2003)

I have found these core conditions useful with people in various stages of long-term and terminal illness. Rogers (2003) rejected the medical mode of making specific diagnosis or finding pathologies to be cured. Instead the therapy is based on being with people in ways that release their own capacity for well-being and contentment.

People can generally understand this but struggle to see how it works when brain function appears to be deteriorating or damaged. But, even in the late stages of dementia, people have capacity to connect with what feels good, in ways we might not have expected. The old medical view used to be that nothing could be done for people with dementia other than attending to basic physical needs and safe-keeping. Thankfully new medical views and increased awareness show that people with dementia can still make connections and communicate preferences.

How to have positive interactions and have a life worth living are factors we are learning through dementia care. The creativity helps us communicate beyond words and share joyfulness. The BICEPS elements for connecting are for all carers. Practice of the basic principles developed by Rogers, combined with creativity and self-awareness is a powerful combination for improving quality of life.

For example, Mrs P. had appeared aloof to many people. They perceived her refusal to join in as a rejection and as a sign that she did not like people. Carers around her responded from a position of defensiveness or misunderstanding, which made it difficult to see her gifts, strengths and needs. Eric and Mr Davis had different issues, but similar experiences of being excluded, because people were not sure how to work with them. It does not have to be that way.

I listened to Kate Swaffer present at the International Conference of Alzheimer's Disease in London in 2012. Kate lives the diagnosis of dementia. This was her request:

Value us… We may not talk, but we feel… Work with us, not for us. (Swaffer 2012)

CHAPTER 3

He Closes His Eyes
When I Am Near

Changes in Relationship

Harold is a young man with a form of dementia that has significantly progressed. His wife spends as many hours a day as she can with him in the care home. They sit and listen to the radio or share a crossword puzzle. Over the years I have been fortunate to witness the dedication of family members supporting their partner or parent. Harold's wife, like many relatives, searches for glimpses of the person she used to know, and sighs when he is not there.

We cannot underestimate the level of distress a carer feels when all their efforts to engage are met with a blank stare or tightly closed eyes. The carer can offer an array of choices such as doing different activities or being in a quiet space. The choices may appear person-centred – and they are genuine choices – but not one of them offers what the person with dementia might want…a full recovery, or less confusion, or to go home.

I acknowledge this with Harold. I tell him I know the offers we present him must seem very flimsy. He glances at me, then resumes staring ahead. It is hard to know what Harold understands, but I get the sense he is all hearing and fully present. I hold up a bright puppet. He grimaces. Or maybe it is a smile. Harold's facial expressions can be difficult to read.

'This might look like a simple puppet,' I say, 'but it took some figuring out to make something this flexible.'

For a few minutes we work together in silence. He turns to look at me and seems to open his mouth to speak, but there are no words, and I do not recognise the mouth shapes. Harold was diagnosed many years before with dementia with Lewy bodies (DLB). The condition includes stiffening of body and facial muscles. Facial expressions can freeze, or appear mask-like, as happens in Parkinson's disease. Movements are difficult, because tiny particles of protein in the brain's nerve cells block the flow of important chemical messengers.

Harold could be telling me to go away for all I know, but when I look into his eyes, I find myself nodding. He nods in return. We have agreed on something that has no words. There is empathy and congruence in the connection. Yet the meaning is inexplicable. It just feels peaceful.

Moments later he shuts his eyes as tightly as possible. This shutting out, shutting down, closing off from the carer or closest relative seems a common experience. Relatives describe the acute pain that such behaviour causes them. The hurt can feel palpable when witnessing the exchange. This behaviour may be fleeting or become a habitual response to someone, and can be due to a number of reasons.

One explanation proffered is that the person with dementia cannot recall who the relative is. They may detect only that this person seriously expects something from them. They do not know what that is, or they feel it is an impossible demand, so they cut off as a defence. The person with dementia may not realise the pain this causes, because they are busy preserving themselves.

Other relatives feel that the person with dementia is fully aware of the pain they cause, and that they do it to convey their own feelings of despair, pain and resentment. As humans we often let other people know just how bad something feels. Family members or long-term carers are sensitive to the distress, because they feel it too, but do not always know how to deal with it.

This chapter explores ways in which relationships change between people who are caregivers and people who receive care. Knowing how to negotiate these changes through creativity can lead to more joyful connections. Puppetry, from the technical making of puppets through to the make-believe world, is one way to connect. The use of maps and metaphors can be effective for understanding changes that have profound emotional impact.

Being given a diagnosis of dementia at any age is tough to deal with. For some, the diagnosis and consequent events are their worst nightmare. Other people describe a sense of relief that they no longer have to pretend they are all right. Either way, it can be useful to understand common experience. Millions of informal, unpaid carers provide the majority of care around the world for people with dementia (World Health Organization and Alzheimer's Disease International 2012).

Spouses are the main carers, followed by adult children, daughters and sons-in-law, and friends. Most family carers take on the role because they love the person they care for. In a European study of approximately 6000 family members caring for an older adult, more than half (57%) identified love and affection as their motivation for being a carer. Another 28 per cent were motivated by either a sense of duty or personal obligation; 3 per cent felt they had no choice (Lamura *et al.* 2008).

But not every person knows what he or she is agreeing to when promising to love and care 'in sickness', or when offering to help a parent. As one relative describes: 'I didn't ask to be a carer. I just found myself being one. It went on for years without a break.'

Peter, who was diagnosed with dementia with Lewy bodies some seven years earlier, is in a care home for respite breaks. He is in the living room at the time of a creative workshop. Staff seem really pleased to see him. They have been concerned about his mental health, because he has become more withdrawn and isolated.

We do not know each other, and the only expectation I have is that we will make a connection. I explain to him, and to his carers, that there is no pressure to do anything. The purpose is to find out what Peter would prefer to do, or not do, but that does not have to happen today.

My first task is to 'tune in' to Peter. This is an important process described more fully in Chapter 4. It requires practice to be free from assumptions or prior knowledge of a person, to offer unconditional positive regard. It is probably one of the hardest things for family members to do because they have such long histories and complex interactions. People interpret other people's behaviours and assume they know their intentions and motivations.

When Peter is seen in the living room, his carers assume he is there because he wants to be part of the action. As they believe this, the staff interact with Peter from that position. They urge him to look at the objects I have brought. They are keen that he participates, because they think this is what he wants. Their eagerness for him to engage, to respond, to show any sign at all, becomes overwhelming.

Peter suddenly brushes the objects off the table, and speaks rapidly. He hurls a barrage of sounds. No words, but the meaning is clear. Peter does not want to be forced to engage. The majority of staff walk away looking disappointed. His main carer picks up the pieces, apologising to me for his behaviour, explaining he did not mean to do it. And so the assumptions continue.

A little while later the carer and I sit either side of Peter, who stares straight ahead. The carer keeps asking him if he can remember significant moments they have shared. It is clear the carer is very fond of Peter. He wants Peter to feel good. Maybe he wants to show they have a great relationship, to affirm that nothing has changed. Maybe he wants Peter to be seen as the friendly man he usually is.

But there is a growing tension in Peter's body, and I know it is time to change the subject. The well-intentioned questions are causing Peter to feel uncomfortable. I pick up a puppet dog and start sniffing around Peter's feet. Peter gives me such an almighty glare, that I spontaneously burst out laughing. He breaks into laughter too – a whole body laugh, without much sound.

Something has shifted. The creative interaction has broken the tension, but it feels like time to be real. I ask Peter how long he has been in the care home. His carer answers for him. This is understandable because Peter has great difficulty speaking, and the carer is trying to be helpful. I am told the story of Peter, about his years of struggling with the disease. Peter laughs.

'Sometimes I think he understands more than I think he does,' says his carer.

I agree that is bound to happen sometimes. Peter laughs again. His body is a little more relaxed. His face has, for the moment, lost its painful looking contortions.

'When communication is unclear, the clues might be misinterpreted,' I say.

'Aye!' says Peter, clearly and meaningfully – and we all look at each other.

When Harold shuts his eyes against his wife, she feels hurt. When Peter sweeps everything off the table, his carers feel disappointment. Everyone involved is upset. Harold and Peter may be defending themselves against great expectations, or displaying their anger and frustration about their experiences of the illness. The pain that people experience can be difficult to talk through.

One man diagnosed with dementia described feeling profoundly sad for his wife. Every time he saw her, he felt her sadness and loss. He said he found it increasingly difficult to be with her, because he felt so terrible for putting her through this. He shut her out because he felt guilty for being a burden. However, she most likely experienced his withdrawal as anger or upset against her.

These emotions run deep and so much can be misconstrued. People often do not know where to begin, or how to express themselves. Sometimes making assumptions or trying to force a sense of normality feels easier than talking about things. But if the assumptions are negative, people miss great opportunities to share love. A similar thing happens when a carer becomes trapped in the feelings of loss for the person they once knew. But all these feelings are part of a huge process.

One view of the process is called 'Becoming Strangers', described by Wuest, Ericson and Stern (1994). It explains how Canadian family caregivers and care-receivers interact with each other along a continuum from Intimacy to Alienation. Alienation occurs after increasing detachment, at which point, a person being cared for may move into a care home. The study shows people pass through areas Wuest *et al.* call 'Dawning', 'Holding On' and 'Letting Go'. I like to view this in terms of a map (see Figure 2). We can explore some of the features of each area in more detail.

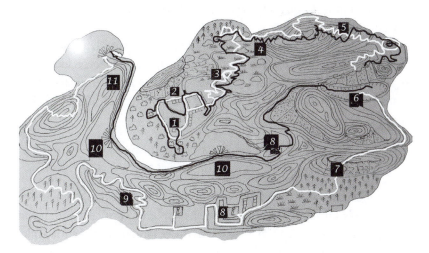

Key: 1. Together 2. Dawning 3. Tensions 4. Holding on 5. The big ask
6. Letting go 7. Alienation 8. Support 9. Inner work
10. Wonderments 11. Reconnecting

Figure 2 The journey of becoming reconnected

Through the ideas and experiences over the years, I have considered that this map goes beyond alienation, towards a place of wonderment. I call this part of the journey 'Becoming Reconnected'. The reconnection does not lead us back to the intimacy of the original relationship described by Wuest *et al.* (1994). It is about connecting through the creativity and joy in the moment of now. This can sound impossible for carers who are running out of energy. But nothing drains a person of energy more quickly than feeling powerless.

This map is a practical tool that offers metaphorical reference points, and helps people see possible routes. It is important to remember that any map is representative. A map is not the same as the experience of walking the actual terrain, but it helps us feel less lost.

Sometimes the beginning of a journey into dementia is not clearly defined. Before a diagnosis is made, it is common for people to consider all sorts of possible reasons for changes in behaviour or memory loss. Indeed many changes can be due to factors such as stress, grief, physical pain, loss of role, infection, a series of disappointments, negative thought patterns and traumatic events. In such cases, when a person feels more settled and optimistic about life, his or her cognitive functions return. Explaining away odd remarks and quirky behaviour may continue for years.

As George and his daughter sandpaper the wooden parts of a puppet, we talk about the early part of their journey. George looks at a bigger version of the map shown here. He was a keen hill-walker and points out the steep contours of the first hills (the holding hills). His daughter feels they have moved on from there.

> '*I think we're here, Dad,' she says, as she points to a place between holding on and letting go, 'but we've climbed a few hills to get here, haven't we?'*

People may have different metaphors for their experiences, such as lost in the woods, all at sea, stranded on the beach or on rocky ground. It can be helpful to create your own maps with the person with dementia. Take a large sheet of paper, and draw your journey, the way you experience it, and where you would like it to go. You could use magazine images of woodland, fields, rivers, sea, gardens, wilderness, volcanoes, mountains, viewpoints, parks and so on to indicate different parts of the journey. Some people like to add weather condition symbols for effect!

Three years earlier George and his daughter were stranded. George's behaviour was worrying, but he would not speak about it. He left bath water running; he accused people of hiding his glasses; he argued in the post office when they refused to give him cash in exchange for the bus pass he presented, instead of his pension book.

This early part of the expedition can be hazardous. People who are experiencing memory losses do all they can to retain autonomy. This apparent denial of a problem is called anosognosia. However, the majority of people I have met are not in denial. They know very well there is something wrong. They barely speak about it because they are in a fierce battle to remain independent.

As MacQuarrie (2005) says, there is a tension between the desire to remain an independent agent, in charge of your own life, while other things undermine a sense of competence. So the person simultaneously acknowledges they have a problem, while fiercely resisting anything that might seem disempowering. In MacQuarrie's (2005) study, some people felt that their carers were bullying them into seeing a doctor, or they perceived offers of help as threats against their independence: 'some acts of care, no matter how well meaning were interpreted by the recipients of care as a diminishment of their person-hood' (MacQuarrie 2005, p.432).

The caregiver and care-receiver may cover up problems. This is not explicitly agreed, but somehow they maintain an illusion that all is well to other people. The caregiver, who sees the personal struggle for autonomy, tries to protect their relative. This can cause an enormous strain because people outside the immediate family may not realise the extent of the problems. But this period is an important time, as the implications of what is happening begin to be recognised. People need time to take it all in.

The ground looks safe and solid, but those experiencing difficulties know they are close to treacherous marshlands. George's daughter felt unable to ask for help. In fact she sometimes thought George was just being a mean-spirited old man, or that somehow she had failed him. People describe the shock they feel when a person they love suddenly stops trusting them, or hurts them. Relationships can be very tricky to negotiate and talk about. After diagnosis, people wish they had been more patient, or understood more about the illness, but everyone does the best they can.

The point of diagnosis brings mixed feelings. An important point to remember is that each person is far greater than any label of Alzheimer's disease, or Lewy bodies, fronto-temporal, vascular or any other form of dementia. The diagnosis offers a general indication about what might happen. The labels can help us understand overall patterns, such as the slow, gradual decline of Alzheimer's disease, or the sudden dip followed by a long level period in vascular dementia. But each experience is unique.

Carers also have individual strengths and boundaries. They often go further than they know how to. The point of diagnosis can trigger a grieving process. Carers may already have been feeling the loss of the relationship. Some carers consider severing ties due to behaviour problems, but feel obligated to stay after the diagnosis. This can be an extremely difficult situation; there is such a taboo about leaving someone who is ill. Other carers find they have renewed energy because they have spent so long feeling bewildered that the diagnosis becomes an ally.

While we can see there may be many blocks to talking openly, dementia is not the only issue. There are myriad complexities between family members that prevent people seeking help. Silence occurs because of family loyalty or due to feeling blame for the way a person is behaving. By the time dementia is diagnosed, relationship matters are in various states of completeness.

Carers sometimes express a loss of confidence in their ability to maintain a relationship, or feel awkward as conversations become more cryptic. They are constantly being careful to avoid upset. People living with dementia are busy finding ways to keep managing. There may be taboo words, such as the word dementia, and certain other topics that are out of bounds. Creating a visual representation of these experiences can help gain a better perspective or an overview.

The misty hills refer to 'half-conversations' experienced by some carers. These add intrigue or distress depending on the topics, such as references to family secrets, misunderstandings, secret loves, cycles of ancestral fallouts, stories of expectations and disappointments, shared joy followed by loss for all that was or could have been, or should have been, references to family battles without winners, heart wounds, profound love, misguided decisions, confused roles, curiosities that may never be understood, half-spoken apologies and hints of subjects that can never be discussed.

The good and the bad of family life now mixes with the mysterious realms of dementia. Although caregivers and care-receivers may have realised something was wrong, there is often a long period before this is clarified. In the early stages, as happened for George and his daughter, the caregiver might believe the antagonistic and hurtful behaviour is personally against them, rather than the fight against losing independence.

Care staff may also experience these battles as people living in the care homes resist loss of control over their lives. This is why person-centred care is an absolute necessity. Usually care staff are able to support each other to deliver this. However, the family carer is dealing with changes with little support. To be asked to be person-centred, give unconditional positive regard, love, empathy and joy – all with integrity – is a big ask! Carers do their best and that best will fluctuate from day to day; it is just the way it goes.

On our map, the holding hills refer to the 'Holding On' phase (Wuest *et al.* 1994), which is about maintaining a good quality of life, in the way the person has always known. In early stages of dementia, carers do many things to help the person live independently. Simple memory aids include notes on calendars, notice boards and diaries; reminder notes, such as a message to take the mobile phone; labels on cupboard doors (or transparent fronted cupboards); and medication boxes with compartments for different times of the day or week.

Assistive technology can help a person stay orientated for longer, such as a large faced clock that also shows whether it is morning or afternoon. There are devices that can record a family member's voice, which can be triggered to play on opening the front door, to say 'Remember your keys'. There are simplified mobile phones that store useful numbers, so the person just presses the name of a person they want to contact. These systems can help preserve a sense of equality for many years within the relationship, as independence is maintained.

The effects of the brain's holes, knots and blocks, caused by dementia, include psychological and emotional adjustments. Individuals are not just dealing with memory loss or behaviour changes. In earlier stages, people can benefit from reminiscence work or activities to keep the brain active (which we discuss later on). People in later stages of dementia require a different focus. The stress of trying to remember or of feeling tested is counter-productive, and damaging to the relationship (although cognitive stimulation is still important: see Chapter 13).

The information points and bridges on the map are where people find support groups, social networks, and organisations dedicated to people with dementia, their carers or both. Make a note of your bridges.

Sharing stories about experience is a powerful way of reducing fears and stigma. Knowing how someone else dealt with a situation can help people clarify what sort of journey they would prefer.

The hills of holding include trying to maintain a relationship that is dealing with so many changes. Some carers find the journey much easier than has been described. The gift of caring may be a privilege and life-affirming experience. Factors that make an experience rewarding and enjoyable include how the person with dementia deals with their situation and whether the carer has a sense of having positive interactions. The experience is also affected by the degree to which the carer feels their own sense of happiness depends on how well their relative feels.

George's daughter realises she is letting go of the relationship that she once had with her father. He often forgets who she is. This started a while ago, but he was able to cover the missing bits and wait for clues from her. She describes this period of the journey as the long goodbye. Some people experience it as being in a wilderness, because the usual reference points, by which they have always connected, are disappearing. This can be a lonely time for carers.

If it is no longer possible to have conversations in words, creative ways of connecting become invaluable. Puppetry is one form, as we saw earlier with the kitten, or with the mouth puppets. George and his daughter find that hands-on making activities can be shared comfortably. The focus is on feeling comfortable, enjoying the task, rather than on their losses. If George's daughter tries to relate to her dad in their old roles, George becomes agitated. It may take a lot more practice to move more fully beyond letting go.

Family carers and long-term paid staff sometimes remark that the person with dementia responds better to strangers. Perhaps this is because there is no complicated history or prior knowledge, so the stranger can form an of-the-moment relationship. As cognitive functions fall away, a person with dementia may become more sensitive to emotional vibrations and demands. The demands may be quite subtle, not even outspoken. The caregiver may just be wishing things could be different, or wishing to be remembered.

People gain such pleasure from being remembered. I notice how motivated and uplifted a relative or paid carer becomes when the person he or she cares for has moments of remembrance. It is a natural, and sometimes hidden, desire to want to feel special. Specialness is that sense of being valuable, valued, important, good enough, lovable and loved.

When we feel loved and valued, we are invincible. The fact that we are remembered gives us a sense of being more special than the person who is not remembered. This can be unhelpful and dangerous territory.

That desire to be special can set up competition between family members or between staff carers. Being remembered makes a person feel more important. Not being remembered can be deeply upsetting and unsettling. This is a huge learning process for many people. Carers discover they themselves must be the validation, the love and support they seek.

The person with dementia and their carer may worry about this phase. How will they cope if what they know as 'identity' starts disappearing. But people do cope. People discover other aspects. We explore this further in Chapter 10.

Alienation occurs when increasing disconnection becomes the usual condition. The carer may experience emotional loss in addition to the increasing physical care (help with daily living tasks, personal care, financial transactions, constant risk assessments and vigilance). Carer burnout happens when the caregiver feels unsupported and drained of energy. A carer may feel inadequate, or guilty for being impatient and constantly tired or frustrated:

> Memory is not the reason carers give up caring. Incontinence, behaviour and confusion are not the main reasons. What causes the carer to give up caring is how happy they feel. (Andrews 2012)

Carers continue more easily when they know they make a positive difference and if they feel supported. Each carer has a personal cliff edge or stop sign. It is the place where they let go of trying to maintain the old relationship, or trying to make the dementia go away. If their own physical and mental well-being is at risk, they may need to stop for a while, and use respite care services or other family members. They may need to hand the caring over to someone else.

Paid carers also experience burnout. In one survey Dunn *et al.* (1994) explained that major stress areas include lack of support from other staff, feeling inadequately trained to do the work, and home/work conflicts. Staff sometimes feel unable to live up to their own expectations about how to do the work, particularly if dealing with behaviour difficulties or aggression. Meanwhile care-receivers also have their preferences about the sort of the care they want. Most people receiving care in the world do not get to choose who gives the care.

That can be stressful if caught in an emotionally negative relationship, and wonderful if landed with many of the amazing carers I meet.

The 'Becoming Strangers' journey from Intimacy to Alienation is for the most part undertaken by both the caregiver and care-receiver together. The next part of the journey I call 'Becoming Reconnected' seems paradoxically to consist of separate expeditions. This is because each must find his or her own way to the 'Being in the moment'. The physical location (in terms of where the care takes place) may remain the same (possibly with more support). Not everyone at alienation point goes into a care home. The journeys are, as before, psychological and emotional. The person with dementia is making the transition between life and death; the carer is on a journey expanding the heart and self-awareness.

Some carers need to reorientate themselves. When the person they care for no longer recognises them, something dies. It can be hard to believe that memory has disappeared, disconnected or been covered over. Sorrowful thoughts are common, such as 'Do I no longer exist in the person's mind? Am I so insignificant that he or she cannot recall me? Did I not count for anything? Was it all a pretence?'

We cannot underestimate the depth of loneliness that carers may experience in alienation. The next part of the journey for carers is to become more flowing, more resilient, open and confident. The support is always there, bridging the gap, but not everyone sees it. Some relatives become stuck in the whirlpools of unfinished business of the relationship. In care homes, staff do not always know how to communicate with someone who has lost words and memory. Focusing on the pain of what is not there is a difficult place to be.

Carers may feel guilty for not having done more, been more, said more; for restricting someone's freedom, or being disloyal; for wishing the person they care for would just go away, or shut up, or stop breathing. Carers sometimes feel guilty if their relative moves into a care home. Guilt is one of those emotions that feel unpleasant for everyone. It offers little towards resolution and cannot produce positive interactions. The carer needs to find ways to soothe and comfort themselves; at times this might be as simple as sitting and staring into space, through to talking with friends or other carers; listening to music; walking; learning something new.

Beyond the rivers of sorrow with its eddies and whirlpools is the beautiful viewpoint. Here the carer recognises himself or herself as a separate being. Their happiness is not dependent upon the wellness of a person they care for. And while the carer has been expanding on things they love, the person with dementia may have become an amazing time-traveller.

The later stages of dementia are where people connect more readily through imagination and feelings. They may yet experience rough terrain. However, carers can become more skilful in using creativity and metaphor to be with people. Some carers envisage their relatives or clients as mind explorers, or space travellers. One person's map contained stars and two moons. There are no limits. In talking about his mother, actor Simon Callow described his view of her journey:

> She's on some sort of subterranean voyage, travelling towards death, making I know not what astonishing discoveries which she has no need or desire to communicate. It's as if she were on a spaceship beyond the reach of telecommunications: one can only guess what kind of provisions she might require and try to provide them for her. (Callow 2010)

Moving into a care home can be a positive choice, especially as more care home staff are learning to work in truly person-centred ways. Relatives may become the bringer of news from distant lands; the friend who has some delicious picnic spread; the chap who has a lovely smile; the lady who brings pens and paper for drawing maps; the man with a kitten in his pocket; or any number of other interactions and wonderments described in this book. The purpose of the visit is to feel comfortable with however it goes.

George's daughter describes the changes in their relationship as a gift. The process of individuation was difficult, but she recognises she has more freedom to pursue things that feel joyful, to bring them to George, in reconnection. Sometimes he is most appreciative of her visits, other times he looks at her new creative project with utter disdain. But it does not matter. When they do connect through the creativity, it feels good and easy and fun.

Continuing as a full-time carer through to end of life care requires many bridges of support. This is the time to connect in a different way, regardless of whether or not we are remembered. Although the person with dementia can take short cuts to wonderment, the carer often takes a longer route. Be open to all the support that is there: the stranger who smiles on the street, the person who makes a positive comment about the day, a helpful shop assistant, support from family or friends, and the various services around for people to phone up and chat to.

The journey from Intimacy through Alienation to Wonderment goes via many lands. It is a way of opening the heart to love someone through all their guises, and to connect with the essence of what makes life feel good in the moment. Create your map, build puppets, use animal puppets, sing, dance, paint. Set your intentions for creating a lovely day – even a pleasant five minutes of connecting beyond the personal is a good start. Explore the ideas in this book to discover more moments of wonderment.

Have fun, and enjoy the connections.

Oh the comfort, the inexpressible comfort of feeling safe with a person; having neither to weigh thoughts nor measure words, but to pour them all out, just as they are, chaff and grain together, knowing that a faithful hand will take and sift them, keep what is worth keeping, and then, with the breath of kindness, blow the rest away. (Craick 1864, p.169)

The greatest gift that you could ever give to another is your own happiness. (Hicks and Hicks 2004, p.88)

CHAPTER 4

The Amazing Grace of Dancing Birds

Communicating Beyond Words

Mr Lavern, with poor eyesight and hearing impairment, appears to be in distress. He calls out to God, in a deep voice of anguish. Staff touch his shoulders or ask him if he wants anything, but his reply is either more callings to God, or 'Help me, help me.' Staff are at a loss as to what to do. Occasionally, when his callings become too disturbing to other residents, he is wheeled out of the living room.

This person seems lost and disconnected. Staff bend over him and rub his hands, they tell him he is all right and that he has no need to worry. But he seems unable to be reassured. The next time we see him, his eyes are closed, but he is calling out, as though in a nightmare. He is breathing rapidly and seems very anxious. He is not diagnosed with dementia but has confusion. This may be partly due to having sensory impairment and living in an environment so different from home.

We have two large puppets, Rocky and Maggie. Their heads are bigger than the average human, with big eyes and big red lips. Rocky has big bushy eyebrows. Maggie wears a red polka-dot scarf. They are both brightly coloured, in ways that ensure their features stand out. The people we meet often pick out yellows and reds, but the important point is to use contrasts, a strong colour against a pale background or vice versa.

We sit quietly either side of Mr Lavern, with Maggie and Rocky on our laps. Mr Lavern's breathing is laboured. His shoulders are all hunched up and his hands are fists. He raises his head, with eyes still closed and shouts again. Maggie and Rocky look up to the ceiling, then look at their laps, as he hangs his head down.

He sighs. The puppets sigh. Big long sighs. And 'breathe' in unison with Mr Lavern. He keeps his eyes shut and his body is in tension. A pulse beats at his temple, and he shifts his position. Maggie and Rocky shift on our laps. We are tuning in. The puppets 'breathe' as he breathes, sigh and shift as he does. Gradually the puppets 'breathe' more deeply, and so does Mr Lavern. He slows his breathing down in harmony with the puppets and ourselves, without seeing or hearing them.

This mirroring, which people often do at a subconscious level when they like someone, treads a fine line. It could be seen as mimicking to tease someone, rather than tuning in to build what neurolinguistic practitioners call 'rapport' or relationship. The difference is in the intention, and the sense of growing connection between the people. We sit with Mr Lavern for fifteen minutes. We do not speak or move, other than in unison with him. We are breathing into the moment.

Knowing how and when to do this is a matter of being aware of what feels right. If our presence caused Mr Lavern to become more anxious, the activity must either change or cease. Tuning into someone is a skill we each possess, if we can still our own minds and body enough. It requires time, but not as long as some might think. Ideally, carers would spend good lengths of quality time with people. We sometimes spend only 15 minutes on a weekly visit with Mr Lavern. Even two minutes of purposeful 'tuning in' has significant impact. There is no excuse not to do it!

To the staff around us, it may seem as though nothing much is going on. Here are two people and their puppets sitting in silence with someone who usually shouts. This time he seems calmer. We know we are in connection with him. We do not need puppets to do this, but it is a good way to breathe life into the puppets, to focus energy into their movement. When Mr Lavern opens his eyes, there will be large, bright, colourful beings waiting for him. Even if his eyesight is poor, he will notice there is something different in his world. We take the risk that he might be shocked. We take the risk, because the alternative is that everything stays the same as before.

Another day – another session with Mr Lavern; his breathing soon becomes calmer and deeper. Maggie and Rocky are in their usual positions. This time he opens his eyes and looks startled to see Rocky, who turns to look at him. Mr Lavern shuts his eyes and sighs.

Rocky looks down at his lap and sighs. Mr Lavern looks through his eyelashes. Rocky remains looking down, but heaves his shoulders up and sighs.

Mr Lavern glances from Rocky to Maggie in quick succession. He looks down at his hands. Another sigh is accompanied by puppet sighs. The beginnings of a smile appear on his face. He screws his eyes tight, then looks again at Rocky. He reaches out and touches the large soft bushy eyebrows. Rocky and Mr Lavern look at each other. He lets his other hand hang over the side of his chair, close to where Maggie is.

Each puppet has our hand inside the glove and sleeve. The other hand works the head movement. Maggie moves to touch Mr Lavern, and he clasps her softly gloved hand. His shoulders drop. They hold hands. He squeezes her fingers. He closes his eyes. We stay another ten minutes, simply breathing and wishing him lots of peace.

Another day – another puppet-breathing session with Maggie and Rocky; Mr Lavern opens his eyes more quickly. He looks from one puppet to the other several times. Not once does he look at us. Rocky waves a hand at him, and Mr Lavern nods. Maggie sings him a song, close up to his face, so the song is in his ear. He smiles to himself.

Later, we are visiting another person sitting in the living room, not far from Mr Lavern. There has been more singing and laughing. Suddenly a great booming voice calls out from Mr Lavern:

'Excuse me, excuse me… I want to join the party, but I don't know the words.'

Maggie and Rocky immediately go to him. We ask what songs he likes, but he shakes his head. It can be difficult to remember song titles at the best of times. By singing the first line of a few songs, we eventually reach a song he lifts his head to. It is a hymn called 'Amazing Grace', written in 1779. Mr Lavern sits up straighter and sings the first verse with such intensity and passion that everyone in the room is moved to tears.

> Amazing grace! How sweet the sound
> That saved a wretch like me!
> I once was lost, but now am found;
> Was blind, but now I see.

He indicates with his conducting hand that Maggie and Rocky should continue singing. They la-la-la for a bit, and he booms out the first verse again. Mr Lavern is alive, uplifted and amazing. There are so many aspects to build on now, to help him out of the world where he felt so lost. He is able to hear the words that have meaning in his life. His voice is so strong, so perhaps he would enjoy being in a choir, or singing after dinner.

Mr Lavern is able to see large, colourful things. Maybe he would enjoy large projected slides of animals, butterflies or insects from natural history society enthusiasts. He enjoys contact with soft materials. Perhaps he would enjoy a hand massage or activities involving felt and wool. The possibilities open further once that initial connection is made.

The next time we meet Mr Lavern, we have two large dancing birds. His smile says it all.

To make the connection when someone seems so lost and confused requires trust and confidence in the process. All caregivers need to know it is possible to connect beyond words. Sometimes the connection happens fleetingly, but it usually builds each time. Practise consciously breathing and tuning-in, for a minute, to family and friends. The more we do this, the easier it becomes to focus on the other person.

Working with silence

Although the gentleman in this story can speak, words were not the way in to this relationship. Silence was. Words may not be very effective with people who are confused, hard of hearing, or distressed. The words of a carer are often said from a cognitive position, while the person is functioning on a more emotional frequency. Tuning in to where the person is requires the carer to find some internal stillness. Breathing into the moment.

When I trained as a nurse in the 1980s, the main principle was to look busy at all times. Once the physical care work was completed of helping people (who were all called patients) to feel fresh, to get dressed and to eat (which was then called toileted, washed and fed), other tasks appeared. It was important to sort the laundry, make the beds and fold the sheets (in a very particular way), measure people's temperatures and blood pressure, do the drugs round, redo wound dressings, write up notes and order the new prescriptions. It was not an environment that encouraged relationship building.

Thankfully many care settings today value holistic care. Staff are aware of the importance of emotional well-being and social inclusion (as and when the individual desires). Some staff need help to remember these values, but the majority are compassionate and congruent.

Family carers have always known about the importance of emotional well-being. Without it, the rest does not mean very much. We can never underestimate the power of feeling connected. It gives people a sense of belonging – not necessarily to a group or a family, but having a place in the world.

There is a quality and depth to silent connection, unlike any other. People may take a while to allow themselves to do this, but it can be beautifully inspiring and satisfying. Silent connection is perhaps like meditation or prayer. There is a sense of the sacred about it, regardless of beliefs or faith. Some students of counselling courses find the prospect of silence daunting, but then discover how effective it is for feeling closer to someone, when done mindfully.

Becoming silent is helped by focus on the breath. Simply notice the breath to begin with, then gradually lengthen your own exhalations. Begin slowly. The person you are working with has not agreed to enter this connection with you. So be respectful, because they may not want a deep and meaningful interaction today, and if they do, they might not want it with you. (It is, by the way, OK not to be the chosen one. You did not spend your life growing up, purely to be the sole provider of all things for someone else, even if that is the position you find yourself in, or what others expect you to do.)

Sometimes the silence can feel awkward as both people feel uncertain. The person with dementia may feel embarrassed that they do not know how to engage with the carer, or the carer feels they ought to say something. We are all so used to filling in silence.

Black *et al.* (2009) mention three kinds of silence in patient–clinician encounters. The awkward silence is unintentional (and undesirable). There is an invitational silence which allows a moment to reflect. Compassionate silence is the one we are aiming for. This is where the silence is shared comfortably, and a sense of compassion is present.

> In compassionate silences, clinicians can find that the silence has a moment-by-moment character that patients can experience as a profound kind of being with, standing with, and contact in a difficult moment. This kind of silence can nurture a mutual sense of understanding and caring. (Black *et al.* 2009, p.114)

For there to be compassion in the silence, the carer must be fully present, and fully focused in being with the person they care for. The focus needs to be as free from judgements or distractions as possible. Carers say they find their minds wander into shopping lists, or plans for what to say, but with practice they settle into the space that is 'now'.

Miracle (2007) describes silence in nursing as being a silence with presence, where the person knows the nurse is there, and feels calm and reassured by the presence, without the nurse needing to speak. In lectures, when students practise being in silence, they notice more about a person, such as minuscule movements and facial expressions. Sometimes the caregiver and care-receiver find themselves smiling at each other. This also happens when the person has visual impairment. Nothing in the physical situation has changed, but they are lighter.

Even at this level of practice, the relationship is enhanced. A study by Chang, Noonan and Tennstedt (1998) showed that when caregivers of older people use religious or spiritual beliefs to cope with stress, they are more likely to have a better relationship with the care-receiver, which is in turn associated with less depression for the caregiver (Chang *et al.* 1998, p.467). Each person will have a range of coping mechanisms. The use of silence is one way to gain inner calmness, while creating a space for the person with dementia to connect.

When words are confused

When nouns go missing, sentences sound confusing, as people try to explain what the object, person or place is. In Alzheimer's disease (the most common form of dementia), the ability to name things becomes increasingly affected. This is not the same as brain ageing, as not every older person has this problem, and the experiences of forgetting names are different.

The work of Nicholas *et al.* (1997) shows that people of all ages can usually use clues successfully to help them find a forgotten word. Anomia is the term used when a person who can speak, just cannot seem to retrieve the spoken word. In tests to name images or objects people might be given the sound of the beginning of the word, or a piece of information about what the object does. This helps the person retrieve the name of the object. However, people with Alzheimer's disease are less able to use these cues. They may even say words that are neither similar in sound nor meaning to the 'target' word.

In my experience people with dementia seem to know what they are trying to say. The brain works hard to find other words to describe the missing name. As a game show, this situation works quite well. The contestants (the carers) have fun trying to solve the mystery word or phrase given by the quizmaster (the person with dementia).

Sometimes the word clues are a little obscure. A good example is given by Talbot (2011), when her mum needed help. The clue her mum gave was: 'the innards have gone up the long ones', which turned out to mean she could not reach 'the handkerchief up her sleeve'.

One man I worked with expressed his desire for an 'Upsy-daisy'. Upsy-daisy is an old phrase used by mothers to encourage their child to stand again after a fall. Or it is said when lifting a child. Having eliminated possible meanings related to standing or a desire to be physically supported, or a desire to go to the toilet, the man pointed at his wrist. He then made a snoring sound. His 'Upsy-daisy' turned out to mean he wanted an alarm clock to wake him up in the morning.

Many phrases make sense when we understand the context. All nouns are just representations of something anyway. A noun is not the 'actual' thing. Individual reference points and meanings enable us to make successful word connections. The problem is that we may not share the same references, so the words may seem way off target. The extent to which people try to express themselves is truly humbling when we see how ingenious the clues are.

We have a much better chance of understanding the words if we share the same culture, context, time frame or imagery as the person with dementia. The phrases below are some of the clues to nouns that people have given to carers (answers to these clues are at the end of the chapter):

1. The white box with the drawers in the kitchen

2. The hickory tick

3. The purple cold with balls on it

4. The sticker inner

5. The yesterday's gone

6. The up and rounds

7. The white that the queen sits on

8. The flat noise.

Dismissing sentences as gibberish causes frustration. The words may not be random or meaningless; however, understanding them takes time and patience. Carers may not always be able to work it out. Try making your own sentence in 30 seconds to see how you can describe 'house' (without using the words home, room, window or roof) or the word 'jar' (without using the words lid, jam or glass).

Anxiety makes the task more difficult. Stress is known to disturb concentration levels and affect short-term memory. A chemical messenger (hormone) called cortisol is released when we are under stress. It helps the body prepare for 'fight or flight' by generating new energy. It triggers tissues to turn into glucose and diverts energy into the muscles and heart, away from the digestive system and away from the brain. When stress is reduced, the body is usually able to rebalance itself.

Long or frequent periods of stress mean that a higher level of cortisol is released. Many studies of the brain, including those by Lupien *et al.* (2005), show that high levels of cortisol are associated with problems with memory and cognitive performance. Finding ways to reduce stress is so important for well-being.

The brain contains many folds. The folds ensure that different parts of the brain are close together, so they can connect quickly. For example, memories connect with feelings, senses, language and meaning in the temporal lobe (the limbic or middle part of the brain either side of your head). We can retrieve a memory by noticing a smell or a song or a feeling that it is connected to.

Inside the brain, on an inner fold, deep in the temporal lobe is the hippocampus. Imagine the shapes of two seahorses lying sideways, one in the right part of the brain, one in the left, and their tails almost joined in the middle – each one is a hippocampus (from the Greek for horse and sea monster). This part of the brain organises where memories are stored, and how they can be retrieved. It sorts out the laying down of new memories and which emotions or senses they are connected with. Any interruption here – which happens with stress and with Alzheimer's disease – has a noticeable effect.

People struggling to express their words or memory need reassurance. Even if the carer is unable to understand the person, they can help reduce stress. Carers can show respect and appreciation for the words. Humour helps, where possible. The carer can also move beyond words, into silent connection, or use body language and gestures.

Some people with a diagnosis of dementia find picture communication resources useful. There are many wordless travel phrase books that have clear images for communicating beyond words. Communication picture boards can also be purchased.

If possible make your own communication book. I have found these more effective with people with profound and multiple learning disability as well as people for whom speech has become difficult. Use real photographs of items, places, people, foods, drinks, furniture, clothes and so on relevant to your lives. This makes the communication more personal than the usual cartoon images.

Another point to remember is that people with dementia who used to read and write often still can. Make use of paper and pens.

Body language and puppet emotions

In the 1960s Mehrabian (2009) created a formula showing how feelings and attitudes are conveyed. The tone of voice or vocal expression is five-and-a-half times more important than the actual words used. And facial expression has one-and-a-half times more impact than vocal expression. This is important to remember when dealing with distressed behaviour in Chapter 5.

Vocal expression (intonation, pitch, loudness) is a major way for people who are sighted or blind to understand what the speaker means. Body language also conveys feelings, personal views or preferences. If we want to express practical information or directions, we probably need a combination of words (written or verbal), images and physical gestures or sign language.

We know when we resonate with someone. We know whether we like a person or not, partly through our sensing of who they are, and partly through reading their body language. The way a person stands can be confrontational or friendly. Eye focus and movements convey understanding, humour, interest, sadness, anger or love.

Tapping fingers may convey irritation, impatience or boredom, but can also be a point of connection, as it was with Nora and her puppet (in Chapter 10). The posture of a body conveys excitement, stress, shyness, confidence or attention. Some signs are very subtle, particularly in later stages of dementia, such as the quick glance by Harold, or the lifting of one finger in acknowledgement of a visitor. These small movements can be as powerful as the tiniest head movement of a puppet.

Puppets and clowns are experts at communicating emotions without words. The most profoundly insightful training I experienced was not the years of nursing, counselling or teaching, but a clowning and mime course. The clown explores human vulnerability and re-presents the dramas and emotions authentically, yet humorously. This is a subtle form of clowning and mime that transfers well to puppetry.

It is such a gift to be able to take a human emotion such as anger, guilt, loneliness, depression, fear, envy or confusion and turn it into something people can comfortably laugh about. The puppeteer needs to focus energy into the puppet and not be too concerned about whether the person with dementia is being attentive. As with connecting in silence, the process may be a few minutes over several sessions, to build rapport and share joyful interactions.

There are many short scenarios based around emotions, which people seem to enjoy. I use this one with a glove puppet if there appears to be little engagement with anyone or anything. Create a glove or hand puppet (see appendices), and try out this scenario:

A curiosity scene to explore the emotions of fear and courage

The first task is to place an object in view of the person. It could be an object that has properties of movement, such as a feather that can float, or a ball or tube that can roll.

The object catches the attention of the puppet. He points and looks at it. He continues pointing at the object, while looking at the person, enticing him or her to look at the object too. (It does not matter whether or not the person looks; stay with the life and joy of the puppet.)

The puppet becomes more engrossed in the object. He looks at it from different angles, including from above and below. He gets ever closer. At some point he reaches out and almost touches the object but suddenly withdraws. He moves away. He might even hide. However, the puppet is curious and finds he cannot stop looking at this object. He creeps closer again.

The object has a particular property that offers a surprise to the puppet when he finally has the courage to touch it. I am often fascinated by the person's reaction, whether or not they have dementia. People know the property of a feather or a ball, yet they become so captivated by the puppet's curiosity and naivety that they also appear completely surprised by the movement.

The point of these little scenarios is to make a connection that is effortless and enjoyable. Finding the magic or the extraordinary in the ordinary is about being present in the moment. Words are not necessary.

There is meditative quality to puppeteering where the breathing, the puppet, the audience member and flow of creative energy becomes one.

When working with people who are blind, and who have dementia, the use of music, rhythm and touch can be incorporated into puppetry connections. One example is Mary, who enjoyed creating a glove puppet that she could make dance. The puppet had long woollen hair and a large floaty silk skirt. Mary could not see these, but she felt them, and she completely understood the joy the puppet brought to others when she made it dance to music she loved.

Another example is of a gentleman who was helped to make a soft-bodied puppet that had long legs. The word 'spidery' was used when describing it. We made spider-like movements with our hands. Whenever we met, he made that movement with his fingers on my hand, and I did the same in return. It was our sign and a remembrance. A signifier.

When communication is difficult, it is good to remember that words are not everything. We can communicate in so many other ways. Of course words can inspire, motivate, clarify, unify, explain, describe, name and help us understand – but they are not the only means we have. We just need a little faith and willingness to try things out. We can experiment and build confidence to work with silence, emotions, movement and puppetry.

Answers to the clues

1. The white box with the drawers in the kitchen – fridge or freezer

2. The hickory tick – clock

3. The purple cold with balls on it – a purple cardigan with round buttons (the lady was cold)

4. The sticker inner – knife (or fork)

5. The yesterday's gone – today

6. The up and rounds – helicopter

7. The white that the queen sits on – a white high chair for a baby girl to sit in for her dinner

8. The flat noise – a flat screen television.

CHAPTER 5

Rocky, My Friend

Connecting in Times of Distress or Conflict

Keith is walking up and down the hallway. He is not responding to the carer calling his name. It is as though he does not hear or see anyone. At one point he bumps into another resident and swears at them. He becomes more anxious in his movements and pats his body all over, as though trying to feel for something. He searches in his trouser pockets, and pulls at them. They are empty.

A carer calls his name again, anxious about Keith's meal getting cold on the table. He calls more urgently to Keith, and walks towards him. But Keith speeds up in the other direction and is swearing louder. The carer realises he is escalating Keith's anxiety, so returns to the dining room. He puts Keith's meal in the oven to keep it warm.

Keith slows down again, which suggests he is aware that the carer is no longer following him. After a while he comes to a standstill in the middle of the long hallway. Another carer comes out of a room and lets Keith know it is dinnertime now. She is very calm and friendly, but Keith seems startled by her, and becomes agitated again, waving his hands around and swearing. The carer says she is going to the dining room and he is welcome to come along too. She walks away. Keith does not follow, he is turning in circles on the spot.

Then he sees Rocky.

'Excuse me,' says Keith as he waves his hands at chest height. 'You look like you can help.'

He is talking to a big bright pink face, with large bushy eyebrows, wearing a trilby, and a little suit, sitting on the arm of a puppeteer.

Rocky, the mouth puppet, responds to Keith with his usual confident gusto.

'Sure, I can help! Anything you want, I'm your man, just let me know.'

Keith sidles up closer to Rocky, staring at the big ping-pong ball eyes.

'It's just I don't know anyone round here…well I know myself…well, I think I know myself… I can't be sure…it's all a bit strange around here… I don't know anyone.'

Rocky holds out his hand. It's the gloved puppeteer's hand. 'Well, let's start with you…it is so good to meet you, Keith – I'm Rocky.'

They shake hands. There is no definite explanation for what has happened here, but Keith has met Rocky before, and Rocky does have a strong, confident presence. Keith continues holding Rocky's soft-gloved hand as they walk down the hallway towards the dining room. Rocky is telling Keith that he has picked exactly the right person to come to, because Rocky knows everyone. Keith is beaming by the time they enter the room. There is something very reassuring about Rocky. Many carers have this wonderful presence too, where people feel utterly safe. Keith does not explain what he has just experienced, so we can only surmise.

The situation occurs more than once, and Keith latches onto Rocky. It is time for another meal. The period before a meal can feel very stressful in care homes. Everyone is busy and on the move at the same time. Once more Keith ignores the staff calling his name. Perhaps he does not realise it is his name being called; perhaps he cannot see their faces clearly enough to know who they are; perhaps he does not like the stress of the mealtimes; perhaps he is having hallucinatory experiences that prevent him from engaging with people.

Rocky appears and says in his heartily enthusiastic manner

'Keith, my friend, my man. How are you? It's Rocky here. How good to see you! How good that you were here at the right time!'

Keith smiles into Rocky's face, taking his gloved hand. 'Rocky, my friend.'

They set off for the dining room. When they arrive, Keith is happy enough to sit and eat his meal. Perhaps it is the certainty about Rocky, the strong facial features, or the out of the ordinariness that attracts

Keith. Perhaps Rocky distracts him from what the problem was before. Rocky's heightened energy and abundant happy-go-lucky nature make a connection with Keith.

The puppet encounters also affirm what is right. This is an important factor to consider. Individuals may be perfectly aware that things are not right in their lives. They may be in the autonomy/dependence war, or the place of deepest confusion just one step away from wonderment.

Several times a day, Keith may be asked to do something that he is losing the ability to do, or forgetting how to do it. Rocky puppet affirms he is doing OK. The language he uses is positive:

'You were right to ask me. I am the right man. You are in the right place at the right time.'

These assurances help alleviate anxieties. People express themselves in whatever ways they can. There is greater awareness that behaviour is our response to internal or external stimuli, or a way of communicating our emotions and meaning. When a person has brain disease, his or her behaviour will be responding to stimuli that we cannot always see or decipher. Swearing, aggression and withdrawal may not have obvious causes, but something is going on for the person.

In the 1980s the term 'challenging behaviour' was used, particularly with people who were unable to make others understand them verbally. One definition is:

> culturally abnormal behaviour of such intensity, frequency or duration that the physical safety of the person or others is likely to be placed in serious jeopardy, or behaviour which is likely to seriously limit use of, or result in the person being denied access to, ordinary community facilities. (Emerson 2001, p.3)

Psychologists explored causes for behaviours using observations, behaviour charts and interviews. They studied how a person interacted with their environment and recorded what was happening before, during and after incidents of challenging behaviour. This information was used to see patterns of behaviour, to understand what triggered outbursts, or motivated such behaviour.

Approaches to dealing with behaviours that were challenging included reinforcing desirable performance through reward systems. Undesirable behaviour was ignored, or managed through, for example, the withdrawal of privileges. This way of modifying behaviour was based on the premise that rewards for 'good' behaviour increase the likelihood of that behaviour being repeated. It was thought that undesirable behaviour, if ignored, would stop. Sometimes it did. But a new behaviour would arise, sometimes more defiant than the last.

Many carers found this way of working too mechanistic. I recall feeling horrified when I was a student nurse, being told to ignore the behaviour of someone who was clearly in deep distress. The idea may have been to ignore the behaviour, not the person. But invariably the person would be ignored. To do this to someone whose world may be falling apart is cruel.

Behaviour modification overlooked the emotions. It focused only on the behaviour. The internal goings on could not be measured, so were largely unaccounted for. I was so glad to have the opportunity, many years later, to deliver three-month courses on more humane ways of approaching and understanding behaviour.

The behaviours carers most refer to when talking about dementia cover a wide range from physical aggression to total withdrawal. Behaviour may be perceived as challenging to some people and not to others. Swearing, close body contact, terrible table manners, shouting and repetition may not bother some people, but could be highly offensive to others. Another definition of challenging behaviour is:

> physical, verbal or non-verbal behaviour that is perceived as causing problems for the individual, other people or the organisation. (Marshall 1999, p.4)

Person-centred approaches to care promote a deeper understanding of the underlying causes of distressing behaviour. We have already seen how important it is to tune into a person to help calm or support him or her. If we consider the ways in which our own behaviour may be disruptive due to tiredness or anger, we know there are numerous triggers in life. It is not that these things in themselves necessarily cause behaviour difficulties, but they contribute to the tipping point towards a point of crisis (see Table 1).

Table 1 Factors contributing to distressing behaviour

External contributory factors	Internal contributory factors
Temperature being too hot	Fear
Too cold	Confusion
Bad smells	Headache
Noise level	Stomach ache
Shrill voices	Muscle ache
Loud bangs	Joint pain
Persistent sounds	Cramp
Lighting level	Toothache
Flashing lights	Anger
Fluorescent lights	Sadness
Narrow spaces	Disappointment
Huge areas to get across	Loss
Crowds	Upset
Other people's behaviour, words or attitudes	Distress
Television dramas portraying distressed people	Discomfort
	Itching
	Incontinence
Doors open	Hunger
Doors shut	Thirst
Uniforms	Embarrassment
Certain colours	Shame
Carpet patterns	Guilt
Weather conditions	Grief
Traffic	Misunderstanding/misperceptions
Untidiness	Sensory impairment
News reports	Frustration
Something not being available	Lack of sleep
Restrictions	Biological/neuro-disturbances
Rules and regulations	Unhappy memories/flashbacks
Being controlled	Hallucinations
Being ignored	Sudden or chronic stress
Being rushed	Constipation
Broken promises	Urinary tract infections
Broken objects or machinery	Illness
Obstacles	Feeling lost
	Not being understood
	Feeling excluded
	Worries
	Feeling overwhelmed

In lectures on this subject, students come up with hundreds of factors. If you hear people say, 'He was behaving like that for no reason', please offer them a few possible reasons to consider. Just because we do not know the cause does not mean there is not one. One lady scratched her carer's wrists, when being helped to stand or sit. She had an undetected broken hip.

Pain

> Common behaviors associated with pain include verbal cues (crying or moaning), nonverbal cues (rubbing or guarding), and facial expressions (frowning or grimacing). However, it's important to remember that these indicators may be absent or difficult to interpret in a cognitively impaired patient. Those with dementia, in particular, may exhibit behaviors less obviously related to pain that are often misinterpreted. For example, agitation and disturbing or aggressive behaviors are often attributed to dementia or psychosis but may be indicators of pain. (Herr 2002, p.65)

Pain can cause significant stress, which in turn causes distraction and forgetfulness. Tsai and Chang (2004) describe how pain is transmitted and responded to. They estimate from other reports that between 64 and 86 per cent of older people experience chronic pain. This 'slow' long pain caused by tissue damage can cause fear, anger and depression. The brain can usually successfully locate fast (sharp, prickling) pain, but Alzheimer's disease may interfere with the process, so sometimes the brain is unable to locate where a person is feeling the pain. But they still feel the discomfort.

Carers need to observe a person's facial expressions, winces, cries and other indications of pain, such as behaviour changes, or holding the body protectively, and mood dips. The Abbey Pain Scale (Abbey *et al.* 2002) is an excellent tool.

Still ask the person directly about pain. People use different phrases for pain, such as hurt, sore, poorly, ache, tender, sting, throbbing, twinge, spasm; so use different phrases at different times to see which register. People may need painkillers. Frampton (2003) states that pain in people with dementia is under-reported and under-treated.

Older adults with dementia receive less pain medication than those who are able to communicate, even though they are just as likely to experience painful illnesses. (Herr, Bjoro and Decker 2006, p.171)

If pain is left untreated, this has a further detrimental effect on mental and physical health, so it is important to consider pain as a possible cause of distress or change in behaviour.

Interestingly, the Staricoff (2004) review of arts in health (mentioned in Chapter 1) shows that participation in the arts helps people manage pain. We know participation in the arts energises people. Enjoyment means that the neurotransmitters of endorphins and dopamines are firing well, and the hormones serotonin and oxytocin are released. This makes us feel good and the perception of pain may be reduced.

One man I worked with experienced chronic back pain. The analgesics made him feel sick and nauseous. He found it hard to concentrate or focus on anything, although he made efforts to engage in conversation. Initially he was hesitant about trying anything creative. He seemed to hurt all over, and the deep furrows at the top of his nose, where his eyebrows begin, indicated the pain was significant. Sitting with him and acknowledging his pain was the first step in this process. The empathy enables us to appreciate the strength a person has, in coping with his or her pain. Breathing with a person helps reduce anxiety.

Painting was something the man agreed to try. We set the intention (the 'I' in BICEPS) to create a lovely half-hour. We looked at a few paintings first. He liked the swirls of Van Gogh's skies, stars and fields. It was a style he found satisfying as he repeated swirls and spirals in paint, oil pastel crayons and pens. (There is something compelling about spirals once you get started!) The man found he gained huge relief from pain through the artwork. He became a prolific spiral maker.

External factors are more easily changed to suit the person. If we understand the cause of disturbance in a person, we can do our best to create better situations. One carer found that her husband became really upset and aggressive every time they left the house, and again when they returned. He sometimes hit her on the arm as they got to the front door. Being unable to explain his problem caused high levels of frustration and anxiety. His wife assumed it was to do with the changes in environment, from inside to outside, or outside to inside.

It turned out to be the doormat. This was a dark brown mat across the hallway by the door, and was being perceived as a large hole in the ground. He must have been terrified of falling down this hole. When the mat was replaced with a pale one, the problem ceased.

In one care home, staff had the television on from first thing in the morning. A daytime show airing traumatic relationship issues with people screaming, crying and shouting at each other came on most days. This does not set the tone for having a magnificent day. The residents seemed on edge and at times were quite rude to one another. None of the people living in the care home had requested to see this television programme. The atmosphere greatly improved when it was switched off.

Approaches to behaviour – see-saw

It is far better to prevent a crisis than deal with one. Imagine a see-saw. One end has people feeling confident, relaxed, quite happy. The other end is crisis and severe distress and disturbance. Towards the middle, in the area that tips the see-saw one way or the other, are signs and signals that show us something is not right.

There are many approaches to dealing with the signs and signals. Some of these are non-invasive, such as de-escalation or distraction. Other interventions include medication or some form of control. What all carers need to remember is that there is a massive array of preventative interventions to help a person feel good about life, so they do not have to be at the tipping point.

Person-centred care helps support people at the preventative end of the see-saw. This includes positive interactions, expression of feelings, meaningful activities, which promote self-esteem, confidence and well-being. Prevention of distress is achieved more effectively when carers are relaxed and positive. People generally feel better when in the company of someone who feels good to be around. We influence one another.

Rarely, disturbing behaviour can suddenly flare up. This might be caused, for example, by delusions or hallucinations. Medication was a popular intervention in the past, particularly the use of antipsychotic medication. This is still used, but with caution, to treat behaviours and psychological symptoms associated with hallucinations (hearing voices or seeing things that other people cannot see), or delusions (believing other people or beings are controlling you; or that you have a very special mission that others are preventing you from fulfilling).

The medication is designed to control symptoms (and thus fulfil some delusional fears). Symptoms include anxiety, confusion and disruptive behaviour. There has been increasing concern about the extensive use of antipsychotic medication. More recent national and international strategies for dementia care emphasise the need for non-pharmacological interventions.

> Evidence exists that, in many cases, difficult behaviour [in dementia care] can be safely managed by use of psychosocial interventions or a person-centred care approach. If these [antipsychotics] must be used, they should be prescribed in low doses over short periods... Discontinuation should be attempted regularly. (World Health Organization and Alzheimer's Disease International 2012, p.64)

One preventative strategy is to be clear about what is expected from people. The practice of positive phrasing is useful. We might, for example, notice someone about to spill their drink, and say, 'Be careful – don't spill your drink.' The person spills their drink. A positive phrasing could be, 'Hold your drink steady', or any phrase that explains *what* to do, rather than what not to do. The brain struggles to compute the abstracts of 'don't' and 'not' compared to the action of 'spill' or 'steady'. Try rephrasing some of these sentences from carers' experiences, where the person did the very thing the brain 'heard':

- Don't hold on so tight.
- Don't sit on the cat.
- Don't tear that up.
- Don't shout like that.

Positive rephrasing takes practice, but has much better results. In a world of dementia, things become confusing. Our work is to be as clear as possible. Rarely does someone actually want to throw a drink over themselves, or hurt their carer, or sit on an animal.

Diversions

Signs and signals might show a person is becoming agitated or distressed. It is usually possible to find some way to divert energy and focus on something away from the crisis. We each have different mannerisms that convey our distress. These micro-signals (Littlechild 1997) could include teeth grinding, glaring, finger tapping, trembling, clenched fists and rapid breathing.

There is a gap between the signal and the crisis, before the see-saw tips. Use this time to intervene with something that either resolves the problem immediately, or changes the course of direction as shown in the following situation.

Outside someone's bedroom is a gentleman who seems lost and anxious. He looks left and right, then back at the door that is not his door. His hands tremor, and he shifts his weight from side to side. It is known that the gentleman sometimes experiences a major rage where he throws things and swears that he wishes he was dead. Staff are very cautious and treat him with great kindness. He has already been shouted at by someone whose room he entered uninvited. He seems to be deciding whether or not to enter the next room.

'The living room is this way,' calls a care assistant as she helps another person walk along the hallway. 'It's nearly teatime.'

The man looks at them briefly, squinting his eyes, but he does not follow. He is muttering. His breathing is becoming more audible, and he clenches his fists. He may be about to enter his personal war zone.

Two big bright fluffy birds come waddling up the hallway, with as much feeling of joy as can be mustered in their comical movements. The man immediately responds. He bends to reach out a hand, clicking his fingers. The birds waddle more quickly towards him. He touches their bright yellow beaks. The birds nuzzle his legs as he strokes them.

The puppeteer does not speak, nor does the man look at her. He focuses only on the birds. The puppeteer moves the man's hand up one of the bird strings to the simple control bar. Together they move the bar and he watches the bird walk and dance. He is instantly a puppeteer.

Now, two birds and two puppeteers stroll up the hallway towards the living room. They arrive just in time for afternoon tea. One bird leads the way to an available seat, and the man follows with his marionette. The first puppeteer reaches for the control bar as the man seats himself. The birds nuzzle his knees.

The care staff bring him a cup of tea and a slice of cake. He immediately breaks off a piece of cake and holds out his hand to the birds. They slowly guzzle the cake, with the help of the puppeteer's hand. Then they waddle away, turning every few steps to wave a bright orange foot at the man. He settles back in his chair and is still smiling as he drinks his tea. He may not even recall the near crisis, because in this moment he is relaxed and satisfied. It would be utterly pointless to change that state of being.

The diversion does not have to be bright birds. It could be a burst of song, or a sudden exclamation about the beautiful colours in the sky, or an instant party. It is a way of using the increasing force of energy that is heading for catastrophe and turning that towards something completely different. Something creative.

To prevent this situation arising in the first place, the carers could explore ways to help the gentleman feel less anxious. Possibly he does not know where his own room is, and could use some clear signifiers to indicate which way to go. All doors could be painted to be as individual as front doors. He could have something on his door that he relates to, that he recognises by touch as well as sight.

Perhaps the hallway lights need to be brighter. The gentleman in this instance seems unable to see the staff or puppeteer, but can see the bright birds. Understanding what he experiences helps resolve the issue to prevent a crisis.

Escalation

Sometimes the distraction comes too late. If mishandled, feelings of frustration or agitation may escalate and hit crisis point. There may be loss of temper, aggression or self-harm. Sometimes carers and the people they care for become locked in a cycle of escalation.

The carer says or does something that the person receiving care perceives as hostile. The person receiving care responds in a way that is perceived as challenging. The carer responds to the challenging behaviour in a way that the person receiving care perceives as more hostile, and so it continues.

These cycles are exasperated by low self-esteem, tiredness and exhaustion. But they do not have to continue forever. One of the people involved just needs to make a decision to change their response. This may not have an immediate effect, because patterns have a habit of staying around for a while after the condition has changed. But finding a healthier response increases the likelihood of living a better quality of life.

In one care home, the team were at a loss as to how to work with a lady who was persistently abusive towards them all. She had very few words, but they were all remarkably rude. The lady had been transferred from another care setting due to a relationship breakdown between staff and the client.

It is unusual to find a team so unanimous in their responses to someone. There is usually at least one person within a staff team or within a family who has a good connection. But this lady was on the verge of being evicted for a second time.

Staff had been forewarned about her abusive threats. She came into a new care setting, with fresh staff, but nothing had changed. During a couple of training sessions, the team members were asked to draw a square to represent the care home and stick figures for everyone in it. The lady was larger than other figures in most people's drawings. Her presence was strong.

However, when asked to do the same thing, the lady drew stick-people in a circle inside a box. When asked which one she was, she shook her head.

'Gone.'

She may have been talking about the previous care home, or the current one. In a way it does not matter. The point is that she was not on the page. In later discussions the staff suggested they might have drawn her anger and her rage, rather than the lady herself. They had prepared themselves for an angry, abusive lady and that is what they got. It is very hard for a person to change when everyone around them is reflecting back a label, a version of them that is not the whole story. Harder still to change when on the edge of oblivion.

This exercise helped staff choose to look for evidence of strengths and qualities. In the beginning staff could manage only 15 minutes of feeling calm in the lady's presence, but this period extended, and more positive remarks were made.

One day a new member of staff made an immediate connection with the lady and the abusive behaviour reduced. A family carer caught in this kind of pattern needs a break to look at what is happening, to see if they can change their perception or response. Be aware of factors that may escalate situations:

- laughing *at* the person
- sarcasm
- telling off/belittling

- shouting

- mimicking

- getting into a verbal battle

- invading personal space

- turning away/ignoring

- running towards a person

- aggressive body language.

Most of these points are obvious, but I would like to look at personal space. This is, as the term suggests, a very individual matter. How much space do *you* like to have around you? It depends on where you are, who you are with, and how you are feeling. Our body distance tends to expand the less we know someone. Personal space was studied by Hall (1966, pp.113–129) in his rather quaint book about human nature. Good friends and family tend to stand physically closer to us than strangers, but there are variations depending on culture and personal preference.

Being touched on the arm can be comforting or threatening. As carers, we need to be aware of how the person is responding. We tend to do this naturally, and adjust our behaviour to suit. If body space feels invaded a natural response is to be defensive or anxious. This is another reason for tuning in with how a person is.

Be aware that when angry or distressed, a person's need for personal space may increase. In a heightened state of anxiety, the individual is more sensitive and protective of his or her space. Some carers notice that people need distances across a whole room.

However, this is a subject of depth because of the uniqueness of individual needs and feelings. Some people in distress and anger actually need a hug. Knowing when to step in and when to keep a safe distance requires awareness and empathy. Being calm and centred is the way. If in doubt, maintain distance, until you know. In the situations with the puppets, the puppeteer remained unobtrusive until there was a sense of 'permission' from the person to enter the space.

De-escalation

The point of crisis occurs when an individual loses control and behaves aggressively towards self or others. If diversion techniques have not worked, we need to find other ways to de-escalate the situation. This prevents the crisis developing any further. It enables the person to feel calm and safe, and offers them a dignified way out of the situation, to rebalance.

Something to remember is that the person in this critical state of losing control, may be feeling extremely frightened and vulnerable. If on the receiving end of violence and aggression, we tend not to see the vulnerability in the attacker. The person may be in pain, petrified, feel trapped and cornered, or have a sense of fighting for his or her life. If the words cannot come out, and the carer cannot see in, there is a major difficulty.

De-escalation or diffusion is the term applied to verbal and non-verbal interactions, which can reduce the threat of violence and help the person feel calmer. If we can remember to breathe and centre ourselves when faced with a crisis, we have a good beginning.

The four stages to de-escalation begin with the importance of assessing the situation. This is something our brains are designed to do. We automatically assess danger levels, but now we must do it consciously. The first things to check are routes of escape! In any aggressive situation it is important that we do not block the exit route for a person who may already be feeling cornered. Equally we need to be in a position to leave if we are in the line of fire.

Sometimes a carer's presence escalates the reaction. It is difficult but better to leave than try to sort the issue out at that moment. Some carers report leaving the person, to return a couple of minutes later with a genuine brightness and desire to connect in a better space.

When outside the room find a way to feel calmer. You could massage an acupressure point on your hand, in the webbing space between your thumb and first finger. Eden (1999) suggests massaging the acupuncture 'K-27' points. Find these by sliding fingers along the collarbone towards the centre. Feel the end bumps and go down about an inch, to an indent that fingers drop into. Tap or massage these points. Or use the old counting to ten method!

Returning to the room in a fresh way gives the person in distress a different encounter. Or at the very least helps reduce your own stress levels. Sometimes in a crisis situation, the person needs their feelings to be acknowledged before they can shift out of the distress (see later).

The first stage, the assessment stage, is usually done in seconds. It includes a quick scan of the room. Does the person have any sharp or heavy objects close at hand? Is there a safe distance between you? Is the route to the doorway clear? Is your body language friendly or defensive? (Standing with your hands on your hips and glaring is not friendly!)

Stand comfortably, with palms open. Decide how you will leave or get help if necessary, and think this while being as calm and still as possible.

The second stage of de-escalation, the critical stage, is to reduce the anger or aggression. The person may not be able to respond to your words. This is nothing to do with dementia. In a heightened state of arousal, people are not connecting on an intellectual level. Everything is on an emotional level. Words can still be used, but it is the tone of voice that matters.

All the non-verbal clues are being noticed: the firm but caring tone of voice, steady, calm body movements, non-threatening position, sense of confidence and safety.

Feeling out of control is extremely uncomfortable. The person is subconsciously searching for a place of safety. The carer can be that place of safety by remaining centred and calm. If there is more than one carer it is usually better that the other(s) wait outside. Two carers can be perceived as very threatening. This is no time for competition. People need to focus on helping the person find a gracious way out of the crisis.

This stage of de-escalation involves the intention of building trust and connection by conveying empathy. You need to show you are on the person's side. How do you show that you understand the person is angry? How do you let them know you can see they are very upset? These things can be said, even quietly, but often it is enough to be with the person, giving unconditional positive regard, using your body language to be open and friendly. Use the techniques from Chapter 4 to help slow down the person's breathing.

Being there helps the person feel that you are on their side. When anger is acknowledged it usually dissipates. The validation of a person's feelings has a powerful and calming influence.

Carers, who could not quite manage the calm approach, described breaking the tension by joining in with the whole thing; not in a battle with the person, but alongside them. They directed aggression energy to cushions or non-breakable things. This is of course another way of showing empathy, so long as it leads into humour or peace following such tension. It would not be desirable or ethical to maintain a state of stressful aggression.

Another option is using puppetry – either as a new focus, or as a way to express the anger and frustration. This could be done in a different time frame, away from the crisis, as narrative work (Chapter 7). There is something very comical and poignant about an angry puppet. One participant of a creative life story project made a puppet to tell his traumatic history. His script contained rage and distress. However, every time the man tried to show how angry his little puppet was, he burst out laughing. The puppet had such a wiggly body it just could not look serious.

When the anger is diminished, carers sometimes walk away to get on with something else. If possible, remain with the person for a while, because they have just experienced something traumatic. They need longer to feel more stable. If a carer leaves too soon, the whole situation can escalate again. Make sure the person feels settled. It is important the person feels they have connection in calm times, and not just when in crisis.

The third and fourth stages of de-escalation are about clarifying and resolving the problem. When dealing with behaviours and emotions linked to brain disease we cannot understand or resolve every issue. However, as already discussed, there are many preventative interventions to use before even getting to the crisis point. We can see patterns of behaviour that might be triggered by environmental factors that can be changed. We can find out the things a person enjoys doing, and help create more gratifying, pain-free and valuable days.

Behaviours that carers find difficult

Some behaviours in later stages of dementia are difficult: leaving the gas on; walking up the road wearing nothing but a scarf and slippers; declining to use the toilet or wear an incontinence pad, then being incontinent; repeatedly asking the same question, all day, every day; sexual disinhibitions, using explicit language, inappropriate touching or assaulting; hoarding objects such as pens, flannels, ties, napkins or, more annoyingly, plugs!

These behaviours are challenging for family members. People do not wish to be disloyal to their relatives by telling everyone about the dementia. Inappropriate vocalisations can cause great offence and embarrassment. Many relationships have hit rocky times because the person with dementia may sometimes make statements that others find shocking and hurtful.

It is as though all tact disappears, so a person may state the obvious about someone's weight, squeaky voice and smell, that no one else would ever mention. It can feel like being in the story of the Emperor's new clothes. Everyone knows the Emperor has no gown, he is naked; but they go along with the majority 'not seeing'. Then the obvious is pointed out to them, and they all gasp in horror.

Collecting objects can be a major issue when out in other people's houses or in the supermarket. These situations take some negotiating, particularly if the third party regards the behaviour as stealing. The person with dementia may not seem at all concerned about his or her behaviour. Stripping off or hissing at strangers might not cause distress to the person with dementia. However, they may be highly offended by other people's responses to their behaviour.

If a person insists upon having the pen that is attached to the chain in the bank, present them with an amazing pen from your pocket, or something else you know the person enjoys. Occasionally it appears that the person with dementia gets hooked into a negative emotional pattern. He or she responds to the carer's embarrassment or discomfort by increasing it! The carer has to find a way to focus on what feels positive, and get support when needed.

The alternative is to feel constantly drained and upset by the behaviour. The subject of carer's becoming aggressive is not popular, but it does happen. People can be patient, very patient, even more patient, suppressing feelings of frustration and anger, until they reach a volatile crisis point.

Jean Vanier, founder of the L'Arche community, gave a series of talks in the 1990s about being human. L'Arche communities, all around the world, consist of people with learning difficulties (intellectual disabilities) and support workers from various backgrounds, living and working together. Vanier (1998) explained that he had not regarded himself as a violent person, but as a carer he learned of his capacity for violence.

> I have experienced my own limits at certain moments, times when I realised there was great anger and violence rising up in me with respect to certain people with disabilities… In a world of constant,

and quite intense, relationships, you quickly sense your inner limits, fears, and blockages… When I was tired or preoccupied, my inner pain and anguish rose more quickly to the surface. (Vanier 1998, p.100)

Family carers have spoken about the shock of realising they were capable of hurting the person they care for. These are complex and sensitive areas for us to negotiate. It is not uncommon to feel high levels of stress. Being able to share these experiences can help carers feel less isolated. People develop strategies for coping with bizarre situations and can share ideas to help one another.

This is a deep and complex subject. Carers are trying to maintain their own balance, while being in solidarity with the person they care for, at the same time as sustaining relationships with other people. One carer had to deal with someone phoning the police and telling them he was being tortured and fed poison. His stories sounded real because he was feeling all the emotions. The pain was real. The words could have come from hallucinations, or a confused memory of television drama. But they were also metaphors that accurately described his fear and pain.

Understanding how to empathise and to de-escalate situations is important. Stress management techniques also help. Knowing why people might behave the way they do helps us respond better. These learning processes help us strengthen self-awareness for the S in BICEPS.

Movement

Sometimes people behave in ways that are challenging because their movements are being restricted. This is usually done to prevent the person from falling, or walking out the front door straight into a busy road. In the past, people who like to walk were called 'wanderers'. They would be constantly directed to sit down. Feeling that other people are trying to control your life is not always delusional!

Walking is a healthy exercise. It gets oxygen flowing into the brain, and this is a good thing. Carers need to weigh up the risks. Over several years of looking at these issues, I notice there are many risks to physical and mental health if movement is limited.

Bowel muscles deteriorate and do not function properly. Constipation can cause a build-up of toxins and pain, including severe headaches. There may be a gradual loss of bowel movement control, which means more work for the carer. Muscle waste means physical strength declines, and the person needs more help from the carer for all personal care. The person may gain weight due to lack of exercise, which means heavier work for the carer.

Psychological problems of being restricted include boredom, frustration and depression. People underestimate how stressful boredom is. People stuck in chairs all day are at great risk of poor mental health. The sense of worthlessness and helplessness is increased. Some carers find it necessary to restrict a person by putting a table across the front of their chair, or tilting the chair backwards for long periods to prevent the person getting up. These interventions must be recorded and reviewed because restraint can break a person's spirit.

The risk of falling should be assessed in relation to the risk of restricted movement. Check the standards of care and restraint policies. Explore ideas for enabling a person to get around more safely: multiple leaning surfaces, rails, walking frames, clear walkways, good lighting, rounded corners, flat walking surfaces, safer footwear, padded hips and so on.

For people who are at risk of heading into traffic, create interesting circular-style walks around the home and garden. Fresh air and enjoyment are stimulating; this helps people feel more alert and coordinated. We need more befrienders to help people get walking in parks and gardens.

Create reasons to walk – to check the garden or water the plants, to pass on a message, or take a cup back to the kitchen. Creative ideas include walking to read a poem on a wall, or to look at a new picture. Have an evening promenade up the garden path. Or take a simple marionette puppet for a walk indoors. Use creative thinking to promote meaningful activities.

If space is limited, try creating a labyrinth (see Figure 3) in one room, or even the garden. A labyrinth is one path in a spiral or circular pattern. People walk labyrinths for meditation purposes. There is something calming about walking one path. I have used many labyrinths at work, and this is my favourite for simplicity. Use tape or wool of a contrasting colour to the ground to create the path edges. Ensure the path is wide enough for two people to walk side by side if the person needs support.

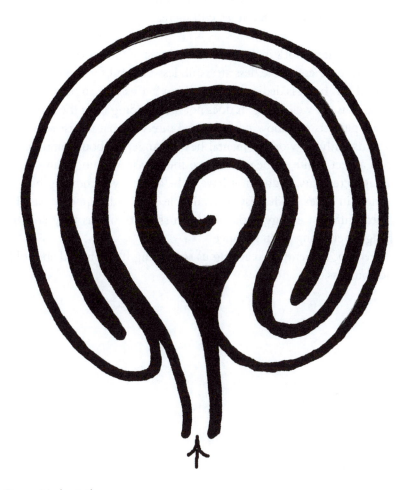

Figure 3 Labyrinth

If a person wants to leave the house or care home because they believe they have to be somewhere (e.g. work, school or home), figure out what the underlying need is. Does the person want to feel useful, occupied, valued or safe? Find a way for those needs to be fulfilled in the place where they are. Chapter 6 helps us to understand human needs more deeply, and this creative way of thinking becomes easier with practice.

Not every carer experiences high levels of stress. People can have wonderful caring relationships right through to the end. Not every person with dementia experiences these behaviours – and not in the early stages. As society develops more awareness and understanding of dementia care, people will have greater confidence in how to live well. Dementia friendly communities will increase positive interactions and support.

When carers work in the preventative area of the behaviour see-saw, life feels more enjoyable, less stressful, less harmful for the brain cells. Most of this book is dedicated to working in this way, so people have a strong sense of well-being. It does not mean hiding from the problems. In fact puppets can show perfectly and directly what the issues are, as happens with my work in mental health. Anger is about wanting life, or an aspect of life, to be different to the way it is. Things can change through creativity. It does not have to be aggressive. Knowing how to connect in times of distress is a valuable gift, and puppetry has that offbeat different energy about it. It can show things as they are, and change everything in an instance.

Perhaps dementia is teaching us something fundamental about life and compassion.

CHAPTER 6

The Man Who Sandpapered the Air, with Pride

A Life Worth Living

Harry's hand hovers above the wooden puppet body he is about to work on. He clutches the sandpaper and makes sanding movements in mid-air, way above his block of wood. Someone else's hand cups his, joining in with the sanding motion, while guiding Harry's sandpaper to make contact with the wood. Harry beams.

'Now I'm working,' he says with pride.

Harry, in his eighties, has a form of dementia that affects his vision and recent memory. It was thought that he might struggle to participate. But his sense of pride, of purpose and appreciation remains intact.

What makes life worth living?

What are we left with if memory and recognition of people and places are no longer possible? What life do we have if we cannot even work out which way up our hand is, or where the toilet is, or what a person means by their words? Some people struggle to see that there is anything worth living for. When I ask the question of students, the gap is telling, for it is not immediately obvious. Our cultures invest so much in memory, memorabilia and making memories.

Sam dozes a lot in his chair. He occasionally engages in conversation, but not to any great depth, and often the same few words. Sometimes Sam slaps his forehead. Maybe he has pain. Maybe he is trying to get his brain to work better. He is of an era when malfunctioning machines would be given a thump or a kick to get them working again. Sometimes Sam swears and then shuts down.

Chris (puppeteer) brings wood, screws and screwdriver, hammer and nails over to Sam. The intention is to enjoy building the frame for a small puppet theatre. If this is not a task Sam wants, Chris can change the event to simply sit with Sam in silent 'beingness'.

However, when Sam sees the materials he is energised. He shuffles to sit upright. Chris shows him the design; a large square shape with measurements sketched on paper. Sam studies this, holding it in different ways, with his 'good hand'. Chris asks Sam to help build the little theatre. Sam replies:

'Why not?!'

The theatre pieces have pre-drilled holes and numbered struts, in the way self-assembly furniture is prepared. This planning and preparation of materials is essential when people have short memory spans. This way more interesting work and results can be gained than would happen if starting from scratch. It depends on the individual. Longer-term projects are perfectly suitable if each stage has a sense of completion for a particular aspect of the whole project.

Sam leans forwards. He holds the screwdriver, which has a magnetic end to hold the screw more easily. Chris holds the wood in place, and they work together. Sam concentrates fully on turning the screwdriver. It is painstakingly slow. Sam's fingers seem to move imperceptibly, but he does not take his eyes off the work. It is clearly a great effort for him and he takes over fifteen minutes to get one screw into the wood. But what an achievement! Sam is thrilled. He leans back in his chair and wiggles his head and body from side to side, in the way one might ruffle imaginary feathers with pleasure!

Sam prepares for using the screwdriver again. Chris adjusts his position, and when they are both ready, they give each other a nod. It is one of those nods that men with a shared purpose give one another. Sam turns the next screw a little faster. His fingers, like huge sausages, feel their way around the screwdriver, which fits perfectly in the palm of his hand.

Mr J., another resident of the care home, comes over. He is clearly drawn to the men at work, although he does not see very well. Chris explains what they are making. Mr J. whistles in appreciation. A seat is found for him.

There is a part of the frame that needs hammering. The nails are held to the wood with small pieces of putty. The hammer is small and lightweight. Many people's arm muscles become frail, with lack of doing everyday tasks. Filling water kettles, washing up, hanging washing, washing cars, polishing, lifting rubbish bags, carrying food shopping, cutting bread, reaching for things off shelves, holding umbrellas – all these ways in which people use their arm muscles are reduced or disappear.

Mr J. is given the hammer. He jokes about building up his biceps, and there is some manly camaraderie. Chris holds the wood in place for the hammering to be done. He offers to show Mr J. the wood, to feel where it is by hand. But this is not the task Mr J. has in mind.

He uses the hammer to make lightweight taps on his thigh. Chris helps him move the tapping hammer to the table, where he hears it. Chris and Mr J. enter a percussion sequence with fingers, hands and hammer taps.

'Well, let's get on with it, lad,' says Mr J. suddenly.

And they set to the task of making the little theatre. We do not know whether the foray into the percussion was a memory repeating itself, or a creative settling into the task. But when Mr J. is ready to begin, he does another unexpected thing. He finds Chris's hand and gives him the hammer. Mr J. takes on a supervisory role. Chris is the worker. They chat about woodwork and Mr J. feels where the nails have gone in, to check how well it is being done.

'Nice job. Neat too,' he says with satisfaction.

Sam finishes the screwdriving, with a declaration that the product is good. He looks around the room. A lady in the corner is making a continuous babbling sound. She is constantly moving around. Sam stares at her for quite a while. He turns to Chris and asks who she is. Chris tells Sam the lady's name. Sam says he will make a note of it, for next time he's passing. He makes no comment about her strange behaviour and vocalisations. He seems contented and relaxed, and sits back in his chair.

The men became involved in different aspects of the puppetry programme. They also take more interest in people around them. When given a pen and paper, Sam does a sketch of a square, with markings.

Perhaps it is the theatre plan. Sam regularly asks for the names of different women he sees in the home. Interestingly, when the theatre is ready, it is the women who use it more.

To begin with staff thought the men would be unlikely participants. But by now, you will be clear that we can never know 100 per cent what is best for another person. Maintaining person-centred principles takes practice. We so easily go with what we believe is best for another, without really checking. Or we assume that what was true yesterday remains so today. We change.

Table 2 Factors that make life worth living beyond memory

What makes a life worth living?
• Having a sense of purpose
• Doing something meaningful
• Things that make the heart sing
• Feeling joy or happiness
• Having a connection with someone
• Having a sense of belonging
• Achieving something
• Having a personal dream that fills the soul
• Knowing each day is an opportunity for living
• Beautiful sunrises and sunsets
• Having a sense of hope
• Love
• Good food and company
• Art and music/the process of creating
• Faith in something
• Enthusiasm for something
• No apparent reason, just wake up feeling life is worth living
• Laughter
• Good quality of life
• Feeling really comfortable

I sometimes meet carers who suggest that the life of a person with dementia is less worthy. This perception may come from a frame of reference that has wide experience of suffering or stigma. People fear forgetfulness, dependency and dying. Working in practical ways with staff and carers is my main focus, so people can 'feel' the work and experience how the principles lead to amazing connections.

What makes a life worth living is greater than memory and cognitive function. People are greater than the diagnosis they have. It is in our feelings that we make the connections. The men experienced relationship through the creative task, but something beyond that in the realm of joyfulness and purpose.

> He who has a why to live can bear almost any how (Friedrich Nietzsche).

Over several years, people have contributed various answers to the question 'What makes a life worth living?' (see Table 2). We might experience one or several of these to have the sensation of life being worthwhile.

As carers, relatives and volunteers, we each have the capacity to help people experience good quality life experiences. There are abundant ways in which we can offer inclusive care that helps someone feel that they belong. We can promote activities that have purpose or promote achievement. While some people do appear to make sudden leaps of transformation (from subdued disengagement to enthusiastic involvement), the process usually happens over several sessions. It is also based on an understanding of human motivation.

What motivates you to get up each day? What motivates you to read this book? You may or may not be clear in your answers. Do you know how to motivate anyone else?

Motivational theory

Motivation is considered to be an internal force or desire that drives a person towards a goal or a level of satisfaction. While we might be able to motivate someone to do something through external forces, we usually need to ensure this has relevance to the person (which makes it more internal really). Motivation is about human nature.

Motivational theory is a big subject for organisations who want highly motivated and productive staff. Our purpose here is to understand what motivates people to increase well-being, reduce depression and reduce the need to behave in ways that are stressful.

Low self-esteem or self-efficacy may contribute to a lack of motivation. Cognitive decline reduces an individual's ability to undertake some tasks. He or she gradually loses belief in personal abilities. It is highly frustrating to have a vision or knowledge of a subject, but be unable to carry out the task. If we pitch a task too high, the person feels a failure. Too low, and the person feels a failure.

Self-esteem and achievement are closely related. The more confident we are, the more empowered we feel and the more likely we are to succeed. Other people's expectations of what we are capable of can be supportive or undermining.

Einstein and Goethe are examples of people who rose beyond other people's limited expectations of them. If carers have limited expectations, and control the environment, there may be little opportunity for individuals to rise above their prospects.

Humanistic theories of motivation suggest people make choices about how to behave, which are influenced by the interactions they have with the world. Our physical and social encounters influence what we do. The behaviour of people with dementia is also affected by changes in cognitive functioning. But the following theory is still a useful tool for carers to understand.

Abraham Maslow (1943) developed a theory of motivation that he described in terms of a pyramid of needs, which human beings seek to fulfil. He suggested five levels of need (see Figure 4). The basic needs along the bottom of the pyramid are concerned with survival: food, water, air, shelter, warmth, sleep and sex. Sex may not be a fundamental survival need for some individuals. The main point is that the overall survival need motivates individuals to find fulfilment. It is very difficult to move onto the next level if struggling to survive, because everything else is meaningless.

Sometimes a person with dementia loses interest in eating and drinking. They may only just be on this hierarchy of needs. A person may not recognise the food in front of them; or cannot see it; or can see it but not like it; or fear choking; or no longer recall how to use their cutlery. Supporting individuals at this basic level of need requires much patience. The carer also needs to use creative thinking to figure what the issues might be, and how to meet basic survival needs.

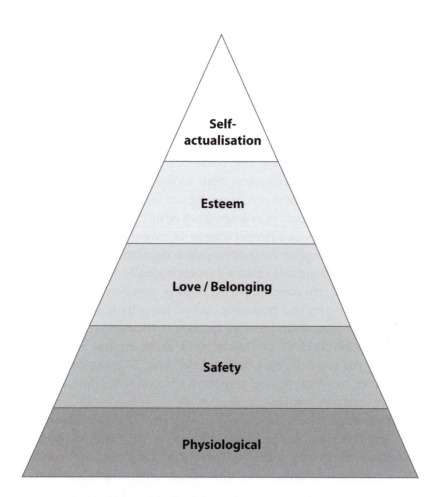

Figure 4 Maslow's hierarchy of needs

When a person's physical needs are met, the person can focus on safety needs. The second level is concerned with security, stability and freedom from fear or stress. Individuals have different degrees of need within this area, and on different occasions. For example, in their own home, a person may feel very safe and secure, but any unfamiliar environment can cause high anxiety.

This hierarchy of motivational needs helps carers understand where a person may be at, and seek to meet needs at that level. Sometimes I see staff doing their best to engage a person in an activity to 'raise the person's self-esteem'. But this has little chance of success if the person is distracted by hunger, or is in a high state of anxiety. The work must start where the person is. We find that out by tuning in.

Once the physical and safety needs are met they cease to be motivating, so the next level is reached to gain satisfaction. While one person loses inhibitions or is naturally sociable, another requires longer to reach the third level. Notice this principle is similar to Roger's (2003) idea that humans naturally tend towards that which is better (see Chapter 2).

The social level is about fulfilling love and belonging needs. It includes feeling loved, giving love, being included, having friends. Some people need lots of social interactions to feel satisfied, while others prefer more solitude. Both sets of people can feel socially fulfilled, but in different ways. A sense of belonging can be met in diverse ways, from hearing someone speak a mother tongue, to having a hug.

Singing sock puppets are great for enhancing a sense of inclusion and social activity. The making of sock puppets is usually done individually (see appendices), but once the puppet is made, group work can happen through the singing and animating. Animal puppetry is perfect for the expression of love, which becomes apparent in Chapter 12.

The fourth level in the hierarchy is about esteem. Self-esteem relates to our sense of self-worth and our sense of being competent. The degree to which we feel respected, or confident in our abilities affects our esteem positively or negatively.

Positive self-esteem increases when we gain a sense of achievement. This also influences our sense of resilience to cope with challenges. Self-esteem is directly linked to feelings of happiness, and healthy self-appreciation. Carers can help validate individual experiences and support ways for the person to gain respect. The desire to gain knowledge and understanding also relates to this level.

Janie shows her dancing queen puppet to her visiting relatives with pride. Later she helps make a cartoon version of herself. She chooses a disco-dancing body. The small theatre fits across her wheelchair. Janie manoeuvres the model puppet. The staff already understand the importance of creativity in Janie's life for gaining a sense of achievement.

When our survival needs, safety, social and esteem needs have all been met, the fifth level is called self-actualisation. The motivation here is to be all that one can be. This is the feeling we experience when all is right in the world. A person feels successful or in complete harmony with life. Some call it a state of bliss, of deepest peace and self-acceptance.

There is debate about whether anyone does actually reach the stage of self-actualisation. But I have met many people who feel they have glimpses, if not days or whole weeks at this level.

All the levels are important. While we can see that each level builds on the one before, it is also true that we move up and down the hierarchy. Circumstances change, and our needs alter. Factors such as moving house, loss of a partner, illness, winning money or experiencing a dream holiday mean our needs change. Not every need has to be met, but an overall satisfaction at each level enables the person to progress.

I think this model helps us see the importance of tuning into where a person is at. When I first met the men described at the beginning of this chapter, I realised we needed to create a sense of safety before aiming for friendship or achievement. A sense of safety was established by allowing people time to get used to Chris (the puppeteer). It may appear to others as though nothing is happening, but connection is building. The next session with the woodworking tools enhanced a sense of familiarity and fellowship at the next level. Movement from belonging to self-esteem was quite fast in this situation.

We can only truly know what motivates another person by understanding his or her experience of the world, likes and dislikes. People's values and motivations change, so flexibility is required to see beyond the obvious. One lady, who was confined to bed, did not eat very much. Carers were very worried about her health. It seemed her basic needs were not being fulfilled; yet the lady was happy in other areas. Although she did not speak, the lady enjoyed company and there was no sense that she felt unsafe. She just politely declined the food.

One day a member of staff brought in an additional plate of food for herself. She laid the bed table for two people. The carer spoke about how wonderful it was to have lunch together and the lady was delighted. She ate more of her meal than usual. The fulfilment of the social need helped her eat her lunch. This process continued. Staff genuinely enjoyed sitting and eating with the lady, and so her self-esteem grew too.

Carers feel motivated when the experience is enjoyable. Without pleasure, work is extremely exhausting.

Motivation increases when people feel valued and appreciated. Deterioration in cognitive function can cause a loss of skills, so we need more ways to bridge the gaps. When Mr Davis (Chapter 2) resumed a semblance of postal duties in his eighties and had the means to walk, he appeared more settled. At the table he was helped to sort the envelopes, postcards and advert flyers into shapes, colours or sizes. He read letters and wrote replies. He had an in-tray and an out-tray. There was a purpose to his day.

Sometimes these needs for self-esteem in older people are ignored. Asian countries tend to respect elders as people with wisdom and experience. Perhaps as the older population increases in Europe and North America, there will be a higher regard for elders in the West. There are several examples highlighted on the Internet of people aged over 80 enjoying life, singing, dancing, governing on boards of directors, travelling and writing.

Quality of life

Dementia and disabilities are not inevitable aspects of ageing. However, many societies still mistakenly regard dementia as synonymous with old age. Dementia can occur at any age. It does seem that as people age the likelihood of being diagnosed with dementia increases, but the majority of people do not develop it. With or without dementia, what matters is a good quality of life.

Quality of life has been defined as:

> an individual's perception of their position in life in the context of the culture and value system in which they live and in relation to their goals, expectations, standards and concerns. (World Health Organization WHOQOL Group 1993, p.1)

Quality of life can be difficult to assess. Quality of life measurements often cover areas such as physical and mental health (including cognitive function), social relationships and activities, independence and freedom and financial circumstances. Banerjee *et al.* (2006) explored whether these types of measurements were appropriate for people with dementia. Findings show that quality of life in dementia does not have a simple relationship with cognition. People felt their quality of life was affected more by psychological and behavioural disturbances such as agitation, disinhibition, mood swings and depression.

Creativity and positive interactions can help reduce the agitation and mood swings. So often opportunities to engage in meaningful activities are reduced as cognitive function declines. Depression is a natural response to life-changing conditions, and sense of loss (of identity, of usefulness, of value). Whatever stage of dementia, creativity is all-inclusive.

Disinhibitions were mentioned in Chapter 5. Disinhibited behaviour disregards the cultural norms and causes difficult social issues for carers to deal with. People might respond in ways that alienate the person with dementia. Maslow's hierarchy of human needs helps us see some people may be operating from the deepest levels of need (sex, hunger, fear), but without the usual understanding of how to moderate these urges.

Quality of life can be enhanced through activities that fulfil the person in other ways or distract the person if he or she is about to enter a disinhibited state. People with dementia (and particularly fronto-temporal lobe dementia) may need more help in terms of figuring out what is and what is not acceptable in society. This is further helped by dementia friendly societies, where people confronted with awkward behaviours know how to respond. For example, rather than take offence and become defensive, the affronted person is calm, firm but gentle, and states the boundaries, while understanding the behaviour is due to the disease. Or he or she learns how to use creative distraction.

For depression, sometimes talking to the person about his or her experiences can help. Focus on what feels right. I asked one man's puppet if he had any words of wisdom for dealing with depression. (The man had depression following stroke and vascular dementia.) The puppet was one of the popular wooden jointed puppets. The man moved the puppet head to look down, then up, then down again. I waited.

'Happiness,' he said.

I asked how to get to happiness. He moved his puppet about more and smiled.

'Like this.'

Physical, psychological and emotional movement are important for quality of life. A group of people with early stage Alzheimer's disease listed the following factors important to them:

- being supported
- maintaining control

- finding meaning

- preserving self-image

- staying healthy.

(Dyck 2007)

What we see in these accounts is that memory is not the major issue for quality of life. Many factors contribute to the sense of having a life worth living. Self-image and identity are explored further in Chapter 10. Being supported, being empowered, having meaning, being respected – these things matter. When people feel good about life they are more energised. They sit up straighter, walk taller; have less fear, more focus, more fulfilment. They inspire people around them. Working with Sam and Mr J. brings pleasure and humour.

Carers need to maintain awareness that they do not pressurise or prohibit anyone from participating. The expectation needs to go beyond personal needs, to aim high, and set intentions for a wonderful time, but then let go of any inclinations to 'make it happen'. Carers need to allow the process and not be wounded if there is no response. Instead, consider what the lessons are.

We need to know when it us who have unfulfilled desires. The person with dementia may be sitting in a quiet world of blissful self-actualisation, while we are seeking the fulfilment of a need to be loved, or noticed or needed.

As we learn more about what dementia teaches us, we may find the criteria change in later stages of dementia for a quality life. It may be less about maintaining control and self-image, and more about loving support, health and joyful connection. It is definitely about wonderment!

CHAPTER 7

My Memory is Like a Dolphin

Narrative Work, Puppets and Celebrations

Mr MacDonald used to be a lighthouse keeper. This piece of narrative is about to be presented through shadow puppets by a group of four people. They sit behind the white cotton screen with their cardboard and cellophane puppets on sticks. The lights are dimmed as a projector lights the back of the screen. The sound is of beach pebbles rolling over each other mixed with classical music.

On one side of the screen is a shadow puppet lighthouse, standing on a rock. The lighthouse has yellow windows at the top, and a red door. A boat appears. It has big red sails and moves serenely across the screen towards the lighthouse. This is the lighthouse where Mr MacDonald works in shifts to protect the lives of sailors, and report the weather conditions to lifeboat stations.

Long strands of blue and green cellophane depict the ocean. Seahorses (hippocampi) enter the scene. Their heads and tails move separately, which gives the impression of them moving through water. Jellyfish, with beautiful tentacles and colourful umbrella fringes, appear. Bright fish of all sizes swim back and forth across the screen. The sea is a place of great beauty.

A diver swims among the fish. But a giant octopus with bright red eyes swoops in. The diver seems to disappear. Next a mermaid with long yellow hair swims around the octopus. She is shaped in a curve, which helps her move quickly in circles. The octopus is dizzy. He leaves the scene. The diver reappears and meets the mermaid. They dance for a while and the show ends. There is applause and the group take a bow.

Mr MacDonald was unable to see the show that was based on one sentence about being a lighthouse keeper. While the group and I worked on the shadow puppets, Mr MacDonald was in hospital. The group extended Mr MacDonald's short piece of narrative with things they knew about lighthouses, the sea and the great mysteries of life. No one knew that Mr MacDonald had passed away. The story felt like a tribute to him.

Another man, who had made the mermaid, also made the diver. He concentrated carefully on cutting the cardboard figures ready for the shadow puppet show. He said his own journey into dementia had made him feel depressed, but he found the puppetry uplifting. It was his decision to make the mermaid and the diver dance together. While the story began with one man's sentence, it became clear that each member of the group had become part of the narrative.

The lady who made the sailboat was truly proud of her creation. The sea creatures were also a source of great delight and people laughed at the angry looking red-eyed octopus. If Mr MacDonald had been able to say more, perhaps the shadow puppet story would have been quite different. His personal narrative may have included seabirds, storms and rescued boats. But perhaps he would have kept the mermaid.

Metaphors and the brain

As in the metaphorical maps created in Chapter 3 on changes in relationship, people often use imagery and stories to express their experiences. These phrases are representative, creative and imaginative. One man at an Age UK friendship group described dementia as a place. He used the word like a noun and seemed at peace with it.

'I go to the dementia. It's where I go to think.'

His dementia sounded like the equivalent of a garden shed, a place to go and contemplate life and the universe. Imagine then if he has a partner or a relative or carer who keeps calling him back into the house, where 'real life' is happening. It is quite possible he would get annoyed. His garden shed of dementia is a place to go and think whatever he needs to think.

Some carers report communication difficulties with the person with dementia. The carer's jokes may not be understood, or the person with dementia takes the meaning of the sentence literally. Some professionals advise being clear and concise with language, saying only what is meant, to reduce confusion or misunderstanding.

It can be useful to practise rephrasing sentences, to give additional clues to the meaning of the words. For example, in a café a man orders his sandwich and tea. The waitress asks if he wants 'salad on the side'. The man bursts out laughing and asks her what she means. She asks him again if he wants salad on the side. He seems really embarrassed, and laughs more nervously.

It is difficult to know exactly what he thinks she is saying. But he is responding to her as though she is propositioning him (the words 'on the side' may be confusing). Rephrasing the question to ask if he would like salad with his sandwich, or tomato and cucumber on the side of his plate, helps the man avoid further misunderstanding and respects everyone's dignity.

Sometimes words get in the way altogether, and non-verbal means are needed. Other times the use of metaphors actually works better than the advised clear and concise talk.

In a study of 39 people with Alzheimer's disease, Papagno (2001) assessed the comprehension of non-literal language over a year. Understanding of the figurative language (the metaphors and idioms) was preserved in most of the participants, whereas impairment to the literal language was more frequent. (Interesting that literal language is usually designed to be clear, but the creative phrases have more impact.)

It seems important to experiment with metaphors. Recognise the importance of the creative and emotional associations of what is being said. The use of applied puppetry is also a great physical three-dimensional metaphor. Is all art metaphor? It is a question that has been around for a long time. Our brains generally tune into metaphors, symbols and parables. We recognise that colourful flags, the music of national anthems and small sticky rectangles on envelopes represent our nations.

> Symbols are profound expressions of human nature. They have occurred in all cultures at all times from their first appearance in Paleolithic cave paintings they have accompanied the development of civilization… They still speak powerfully to us, simultaneously addressing our intellect, emotions, and spirit. Their study is the study of humanity itself. (Fontana 1993, p.8)

Around the world we find different kinds of good luck symbols such as four-leaf clovers; chirping crickets; pigs and frogs; chimney sweeps; a circle; a St Christopher charm; the hand; the heart; and various numbers. We attach emotions to these symbols. The ease with which we engage with metaphors seems to happen inside another inner fold of our brain.

This inner fold is made from the outer part of the brain (the cerebral cortex). I like to describe it this way: use a handkerchief or large tissue to represent the cerebral cortex. Place it over your closed fist-shaped hand (which represents the rest of the brain). Now stuff some of the handkerchief inside the space where your thumb is. That's the deep fold in the cerebral cortex, called the insula. It is like an inner island. You have one of these on each side of your head. (The plural of insula is insulae.)

If you have stuffed enough material in there, you'll notice it has its own folds or furrows. Try turning your wrist so you can see the fold from the other side. In anatomy, the insula has four large furrows, called sulci (Afif *et al.* 2009). This connects the insula to many other parts of the brain. The insula is an incredibly versatile centre dealing with empathy, trust, delight, disgust and physical bodily sensations such as pain (real or imagined). It also helps us imagine how we might feel (physically or emotionally) in certain situations.

Johann Christian Reil discovered the insula in 1796 (Binder, Schaller and Clusmann 2007). The fourth furrow of the insula has only just been discovered, over 200 years later. Reil, who developed German psychiatry, also wrote about the importance of creativity and music in a very metaphorical way:

> music quiets the storm of the soul, chases away the cloud of gloom, and for a while dampens the uncontrolled tumult of frenzy. (Reil, cited in Binder *et al.* 2007, p.1092)

Parts of the insula can be affected by vascular damage, such as a stroke, where a burst blood vessel or clot cuts off the blood supply, or tiny blood vessels are damaged inside the cortex. Some damage can cause a lack of awareness of the other side of the body, called 'spatial neglect' (Golay, Schnider and Ptak 2008). But physical recovery of movement and speech is possible. Individuals have different experiences of vascular damage.

Bert's left side, especially his arm, is affected by a stroke. He regularly exercises, which helps regain mobility and he can now walk. Bert does not say very much; he likes to observe. As he becomes more involved in the puppetry programme, he chats more. His carers talk about a photograph he has on his wall. It is of his fishing boat with a dolphin jumping in the air out front. This piece of narrative is full of creative possibilities.

We create a shadow puppet boat like the one in the photograph, plus two dolphins. Bert laughs as the dolphins jump and dive around the boat on the screen. He talks with a carer about the fish he used to catch: herring, mackerel, salmon, cod, haddock, hake, flatfish, prawns, crabs and lobsters.

On the next occasion he says:

'My memory is like a dolphin, it comes and goes.'

In another setting, William recovered his movement and speech following a stroke. He now has vascular dementia, making him forgetful and sometimes low in mood. William is aware of having memory problems, and says that makes him feel 'on edge' (anxious), in case he forgets something important.

William's story begins with a man living beside the sea. The sea and fishing industries are an important part of Scottish history, which explains why many stories relate to this great subject. Individual stories weave in and out of history, myths and legends.

The story fragment is that one full moon, the high tide crashed waves and rocks around his house. After establishing, through the drawing of rough sketches what the house looked like, the group set to work creating the shadow puppet home, with yellow windows, and a door that opens. They make a man, some rocks and large waves.

However, the people performing this story make a significant change to the narrative, as they ad-lib their way through it. The house is swept into the sea, leaving the man standing on top of a big rock. I turn to William and ask if he wants to change the ending, but he seems enthralled. He asks the performers to do it again, just the same.

'That's it! That's it,' he says.

He offers no further explanation at the time, but seems quite content. In another session we talk about dementia, William and I share the imagery of the storm and the house swept out to sea. It becomes metaphor for the stroke and brain damage. What we are left with is one man still standing.

Metaphor is powerful. In an article about having a metaphor for the ageing brain, Rockwood (2007) suggests that instead of thinking in terms of battle, with all its negative connotations, we could use the metaphor of a series of marathons.

> As our brains age, we must prepare them to resist injury – equip them with good educations, train them thoughtfully with challenging regimens, support them with nurturing environments, and be prepared to refresh them from time to time. We should also recognise that performance can vary dramatically from one marathon to the next. (Rockwood 2007, p.1897)

Rockwood (2007) suggests the most important consequence of this type of metaphor is that we regard the process as something to prepare for, and accept that even elite athletes slow down and reflect on what has been achieved along the way, before the race ends.

The way we see the world affects how we deal with things. Through creative thinking and narrative work, people have opportunities to do so much more than has usually been expected. One man still standing has lots to see, places to go, thoughts to think.

A lot of my work with people experiencing mental ill-health and recovery explores the metaphors they use to describe their situations. Being ill, while on a journey of self-discovery, has a different quality to feeling ill as hopeless damage and failure. Many of us learned to view illness and disease as the enemy. The language used by medical professionals and patients means that people miss opportunities to explore other connections. Creativity allows us to consider the dementia or disease from different angles. Living with dementia is better than suffering from dementia.

Part of the problem about disease is that we are conditioned 'to see disease as something bad, to be gotten rid of, eradicated, fought against, blocked, and beaten' (Jobst, Shostak and Whitehouse 1999, p.497). They suggest that a change in metaphors will help us understand and respond to major diseases differently. Is it possible for us to regard disease as a desire to change something in our lives? This has a different feel to the current metaphors that show disease as the enemy.

While attending conferences about dementia care, I have noticed several military-style metaphors, for example Fighting the cruel disease; Victims; Army of the forgetful; Tackling the epidemic; Aggressive disease. The doctors and researchers are seen as valiant heroes in the war against cancer or the battle against Alzheimer's disease. Metaphors are more than words. They carry strong emotional content and heavily influence our responses and thoughts.

Some people experience the battle cry in a Spartacus or Braveheart William Wallace sort of way. They are motivated to do something, such as raise money for research; create supportive clubs and organisations; take up new challenges to help ward off and beat the disease. Some people declare that the fight is what keeps them alive. They fight for their lives, as warriors, and can achieve great things. We see the Dementia Action Alliance call for reviews on the use of antipsychotic prescriptions; the dementia challengers helping relatives find support; the dementia friendly communities learning how to support people to live in their community.

Other people find the war metaphors alienating. They feel flattened by the idea that their brain and body are under attack, or that their partner is a victim and everything has gone wrong. Some people become paralysed with fear; they make their lives smaller, withdrawing as much as possible. To them, the metaphor about the disease as the enemy feels destructive and devastating. People feel ruled by the soldiers, whether they are enemy or friendly soldiers. They feel disempowered and need a new set of metaphors.

If disease is seen as having a more benevolent nature it changes our thinking:

> enabling people to see that [diseases] are not necessarily 'going wrong' but are, in fact, helping [people] become stronger, to live more fully and with more understanding. Seen from this perspective, depression; cancer; heart disease; neurodegenerative and autoimmune disease; [and] dementia;…are 'diseases of meaning.' (Jobst *et al.* 1999, p.495)

Whether we regard disease as the enemy, or as part of a spiritual journey, may not change the prognosis, but it will greatly influence our quality of life.

Puppetry narrative

Hundreds of people have told their stories through our narrative puppetry programmes. Each participant enters the creative process with or without words, making characters that represent who they are.

Puppets have been used all around the world to explore issues. As mentioned in Chapter 1, touring puppets made comment upon social and political matters. They told bible stories and brought news of events. Punch was a rebellious puppet that in the seventeenth century made stark political comments about the huge social upheavals (e.g. religious revolts or English civil war). Punch played a simpleton who could ridicule the government or even the King and avoid death.

In the 1960s the Bread and Puppet Theatre (USA) told stories about problems in the neighbourhood, and protested against the Vietnam war. They continue making social comment and tour the world. Television puppet shows have used humour and satire to illustrate political or controversial issues. Some of these include *Spitting Image* (UK), *The XYZ Show* (Kenya, Africa) and Quaisar's show *Political Buds* (Pakistan).

These shows are scripted and have clear aims about the sorts of messages they wish to convey. They may draw attention to injustice or power struggles, and help the audience consider wider issues. This is not always the case in narrative puppetry, unless people want to create a definite performance (see Chapter 15). Our work begins with a framework, such as a theme, but the rest is really about process.

The puppet is made with the person, to represent current life experience. Making the puppet is often a major part of the work. From initial designs through to completion, we may discover there are narratives spanning several years. Sometimes two or three self puppets are required to represent different stages of life. Other times the experience is not specifically about narrative, but about making connections.

People gain a different perspective when they see their puppet story. In the gap between a person's life experience, and what they see on the screen (or in their puppet), there is opportunity for a change of attitude or realisation. We saw this with William here, and again with Bert earlier.

Although narrative puppetry externalises the person's story, this is not always a conscious aim. It just happens because the puppet is naturally an external version of the person's story. This helps a person see his or her experience differently. There are many profoundly moving experiences and revelations as the puppet expresses an individual's story on an emotional level.

It is not at all necessary to focus on a particular issue or problem. I might ask someone, 'If you had a story to tell, where would it begin?' The person might be a carer, a relative or someone living with dementia.

A person's narrative might be about a particular moment in time, an incident, a feeling, a memory. Wherever it is, it is a good place to start. Sometimes we work with a theme such as 'stories about attitudes' or 'stories about well-being'.

Shadow puppets are ideal for shorter sessions, and for group work. The puppets are easy to make from cardboard; we often provide basic templates. The lighting has to change from usual room lighting to darkness, so the projector can cast the puppet shadows onto the screen. This can work well if people are given plenty of time for their eyes to adjust.

On the subject of eyesight, quality of vision is important at any age, but is sometimes neglected in dementia care. We should check whether people need glasses, as vision impairment affects social interactions and perceptions. Disturbances in vision in Alzheimer's disease may include blurred vision, and reduced colour discrimination (more than usually happens in ageing) (Salamone *et al.* 2009).

Good lighting is essential at any time, and especially for making the puppets. Before using the screen, we explain what we are going to do. Seeing the puppets on a screen requires the room lights to be dimmed, the curtains drawn, and the projector light to be on. Although very versatile and effective, shadow puppets are not very 'cuddly'.

The hand puppet, rod puppet or marionette puppets have more emotional appeal. When a person holds a puppet of him or herself, there is a sense of intrigue and wonderment. The little version of a person conveys both vulnerability and power. It is a curious combination.

Participants perform in different ways. One man gave his puppet the ability to fly from object to object. Each time a new object appeared the puppet flew directly there and hugged it, then onto the next. At the end of flying the puppet lay down. The man gathered the objects to the puppet, who was now lifeless.

We do not always know what the story means in cognitive or factual terms. But there is great connectedness with the performance. What we applaud is the courage someone has to give something a go; the vision, the creativity and connection we witness. Individuals sometimes repeat their performance and introduce a different element. Puppets can do that.

Narrative and healing stories

Stories nurture us. We gain understanding and validation from stories that highlight qualities of love or courage, strength and trust. Even one fragment of life story can inspire people to find meaning, because we are all stories.

Narrative is the retelling of events. For over 50 years, James Bruner, a cognitive psychologist, explored the way narrative enables us to create meaning in our lives (Bruner 2003 pp.64–68). We retell accounts of our experiences in different ways, depending on who we telling, how they are responding, and how we are feeling about the narrative. Who we are is defined by us as individuals telling our stories, and by the culture in which we participate.

> There is no such thing as an intuitively obvious and essential self to know, one that just sits there ready to be portrayed in words. (Bruner 2003, p.64)

Our narrative interacts and changes as we make sense of experiences, or respond to how we think others see us. We may have narratives that we keep to ourselves, while telling others a different version. The narrative work may not be linear or even about an existing event. But the person's story is an account of something about his or her life experience.

> There are different ways to tell your stories. It's not that one is true and the other is not true. It's a matter of emphasis and context. (Bateson 1993, p.42)

If we find ourselves disorientated, we can gain perspective by viewing our life in terms of an adventure story. For example, a hero in a story usually has some great obstacle, dilemma or major challenge that he must deal with. How he does that through perseverance or love or magical interventions, or faith or help, can offer us comfort and hope.

In her book about gathering stories, Baldwin (2005) suggests that as we tell our stories, we have moments of realisation. We link up with other stories and memories that support this realisation. This builds new narratives. It is a process of self-development. If we did not do that, our lives might be small. Other people's stories about who we are can be limiting or empowering. This is a huge subject, so I am really just highlighting the importance of story in our lives. I have also found that some stories go beyond words.

People with dementia may reach a place where they are unable to remember or retrieve the usual stories about who they are. Other people start telling those stories instead. But any story we tell about another person has something of us in it, our version, our feelings, our meaning, our memories, our words. When a person can no longer remember their own stories, there is often an assumption that this is the end of who they are. How can we possibly know that?

In this work, we find that people who have gone beyond speaking words still connect with stories, songs, puppetry, joyfulness and love. We see faces light in recognition of good feelings. When someone cannot remember how to tell their old story it is the perfect time for making stories about wonderment, enjoyment, mystery and romance in the moment. The feelings are more important than the content. That is probably true for all of us, at any stage of life.

Themed days and celebration works

The following are some ideas, big and small, cheap and expensive, short-term and longer-term about creating stories in the moment that feel good. There are always opportunities to celebrate life. Sometimes people remember things linked to the subject. This is because the physical experience, sights and sounds, trigger different brain patterns that connect briefly to the memory. But reminiscence is not the main purpose of these creative excursions. We are simply finding ways to create stories in the now.

Ideally, where possible, people would be supported to have physical experiences that are inspiring, interesting and fun. Real fresh air, sights, sounds and smells are stimulating. As we move into dementia friendly communities, more organisations will realise they can adapt their existing educational programmes or visitor experiences.

The Museum of Modern Art (MoMA), New York, offers 'Meet Me at MoMA'. It is a monthly programme that makes art accessible for people with Alzheimer's disease and their families. It provides opportunities to look at and hear about the art. People become involved in dialogue about art themes, artists and artwork.

Carrie McGee, who helped set up the project, explains that one of the biggest joys is seeing family members and people with dementia laughing and sharing the art experiences together. There is no divide between the person with dementia and the family member:

> They interact with the programme on the same level… It is a level that is very high… People are less afraid to give a wider interpretation [of the art]. (Museum of Modern Art, 2012)

Businesses and regular visitor attractions offer short tours or mini-talks about their places of work. It is worth contacting any organisation you can think of to see what is possible for people with dementia. Some airports, for example, offer tours, or guidance packs for school parties about how an airport works, which can be tailored to adults. People might like to visit for the interactions or to sit and watch people.

Other ideas include going to steam railways, zoos, parks, beaches, night sky observatories, gardens, museums, spice markets, country houses, castles, restaurants, cinemas, viewpoints, waterfalls, the desert, churches, mosques and temples, fire stations, police stations, distilleries, harbours, school concerts, live music, orangutan sanctuaries, theatres, golf clubs, cricket pavilions, sporting events, choirs, archaeological digs, sewerage works, rickshaw rides, ballroom dancing, famous statues, bridges, railway stations, canal barge trips, sheep farms, cattle farms, riding stables, antique fairs, auctions and music shops.

Many factories offer tours so people can see the manufacturing process, such as: the Boeing Everett (plane parts) factory in Seattle, USA; chocolate making at Cadbury World in Birmingham, UK; Ferrari car test track tour, Modena, Italy; Guinness Brewery, Dublin, Ireland; Haribo Gummy Bear factory, Bonn, Germany; the world's largest particle physicist laboratory, CERN, Geneva, Switzerland; the Santa Claus village in Lapland, Finland; bicycle manufacturers; piano restorers; print-makers; perfume and mobile home manufacturers.

If by now you are buzzing with ideas, all well and good. If, on the other hand, you have found yourself in the land of the impossible, you need to turn around and see where all this is heading. The trick is to dwell in the land of possibilities.

All of the above ideas can be translated in some form or other for experiences in a care home, community centre and domestic home. In fact, people get even more ideas springing from these themes, as creativity begets itself. We expand our understanding, ideas and sense of fun. The following are just some ideas to play with.

Museum tour

In an imaginary museum tour, find interesting objects from around the home and label them. Individuals can be the curators. Examine, clean and photograph (or sketch) the objects. Label them with whatever name seems appropriate. Write a brief description of the article's history (real or imagined) and suggest its age and value. This exercise can develop to giving mini-talks or guided tours about the objects. Create a museum handbook or scrapbook. Add prices and you have a museum shop or a basis for an auction.

Visiting the seaside

For visiting the seaside, roll up your trousers to sit on a deck chair in Brighton, with a knotted handkerchief or sunhat on your head. Sip lemonade and cocktails on the beach at Saint Tropez. Spread a warm beach towel beneath your feet on the busy beaches of Benidorm. Enjoy watching the sea from your hotel balcony. It does not matter where the imaginary place is, so long as the atmosphere of being there can be created. Cover chairs with striped material. Create sounds of seagulls, ice-cream vans, children laughing. There are CDs of the rhythmic sounds of the sea, and videos of waves and sea creatures. Paddle in warm water (bowls); apply sun lotion (moisturising cream on face and hands); write postcards; watch a Punch and Judy show.

Book festival

For a book festival, the room is full of authors. Have a theme or categories such as crime novels, children's literature, comedy and non-fiction. Create book jackets and titles. Cover real books with these covers (preferably books that the person enjoys reading, or having read to them). Read extracts from the books and have a discussion or congratulate the author on the fine prose. Do other book festival-related activities: have book displays; set up a tea and cake tent; invite real authors; invite children to read their latest essay; create paper sculptures; award prizes; dress up as characters from famous books; and set up book reading clubs.

Dream holiday

For a dream holiday, some of the most exciting feelings about having a holiday are in the planning stage. There is a period of anticipation, expectation, dreams, visualisation and excitement as we imagine where we are going; what the weather will be like; what we will wear; where we will stay; how we will get there; what the food will be like; how relaxing or interesting it will be. This entire prelude to the event is important and yet it is all imaginary! Of course in 'real' life we usually go on the holiday, because not going would feel disappointing. So acknowledge that this is about taking an imaginary trip. Many people do this activity anyway, knowing they will not be going, but enjoying the thoughts. Find maps, make lists, explore travel magazines, circle desirable hotels or excursions, make luggage labels, draw up an itinerary, and create travel tickets. This activity can extend to creating guidebooks, writing travel reports, sending postcards.

Bird-watching

Bird-watching could take place in the garden or from a window, where the bird table or bird feeders are visible. Use lightweight binoculars, and a bird-identifier book or printed sheets with the most likely bird visitors. Invite enthusiastic bird-watchers and speakers to share their knowledge. There are bird-watching educational resources such as CDs of birdsong and fact sheets. The Royal Society for the Protection of Birds sell singing cuddly toy versions of the real birds. These also help people identify the bird songs. Production activities could include bird tables, nest boxes, fat balls and bird cake.

Model railway

Who does not like to see a model railway? What can beat the sight of replica bushes on dark green embankments, and tiny people standing on platforms with their suitcases, or sitting on little white benches? Signals and points; tunnels and bridges; rock face and trees. The stationmaster's house and a porter with a miniature sack barrow wait in readiness for the train. Houses with lit windows, churches with bells and sheep on the hills. Apparently Frank Sinatra appreciated model railways as do other rich and famous people: Rod Stewart, Roger Daltrey and Jools Holland. Nobutaro Hara, a well-known collector, has opened the Hara Model Railway Museum in Yokohama, Japan. There are model rail enthusiasts all around the world. Invite them over for tea!

Community links

Use community links to bring news, ideas and enthusiasm into the home. Care home managers and staff may understandably have concerns about health and safety, but these are matters for ongoing assessment, negotiation and risk management. History shows us that untoward behaviour in care settings happens more when the environment is institutionalised and closed. Make use of advocacy and befriending schemes as the vetting is already done. Create programmes where there are always staff around. Health and safety should never be used as an excuse to just contain people.

Local schools and colleges need supportive audiences for drama and singing groups. Do exchanges – for example, create a puppet show for the school, in exchange for the pupils coming to entertain. These ideas can still be applied in the family home, but on a smaller scale, with family, grandchildren or neighbours. Connect with other carers for support to try some ideas. Check available community groups.

The activities throughout this chapter are about transforming environments and making story in the moment. Mark the seasons and festival days. There are myriad ways to celebrate life!

CHAPTER 8

The Etiquette of Dreadful Singing

Singing Puppets

Edna-eski is a large puppet with a big voice who loves to sing. Named after a friend's mother, Edna-eski does not take any nonsense. In fairy tales Edna-eski plays Cinderella's ugly sister, or Vasalisa's wicked stepmother. She usually wears a head turban, which is bright gold with a red flower. Her long skirts bustle as she moves and her mouth is all wrinkled, as she has no teeth. (Her namesake looked much prettier!) The thing about Edna-eski is that she sings very badly.

Today we are forming a new singing group. Usually we sit in an open circle, but today's group is around a table. There is a song sheet for the lyrics of 'You Are My Sunshine', which was recorded by Jimmie Davis in 1940 (Peer International Corp copyright). We are awaiting the arrival of our singing teacher. One or two people are concerned that they do not sing very well. They will undoubtedly feel more competent when Edna-eski arrives.

One gentleman appears to be asleep. He sleeps most days and rarely interacts with anyone. A lady fiddles anxiously with the collar of her knitted top, and then her skirt. Another stares far into space, clutching her handbag on her lap. A man brushes invisible things off the table, and off his lap.

When Edna-eski makes her grand entrance, everyone wakes up. Her tone of voice is like that of an old-fashioned matron or head teacher, commanding and demanding everyone to pay attention. But because she is so comical to look at (and clearly a puppet), people find her character very funny.

A male puppeteer usually works Edna-eski, which is in keeping with the tradition of men performing those characters. The back of her head has a rod, which takes the weight of her whole body. A stick coming out of the elbow controls her right arm. Her other hand is fixed on her hip, so she can appear to stand with both hands on her hips, and peer down at people in their chairs. Today, she is here to lead the new singing group.

'A song a day keeps the doctor away,' she declares. 'We must all sing for our supper and keep the wolves at bay.'

The gentleman, who spends much of his life snoozing, looks Edna-eski up and down and chuckles to himself. She turns to him and declares he must be her leading man in her next film. She holds out a gloved hand for him to kiss. He turns to look at his neighbour and they share a smile.

Now Edna-eski is ready to sing. She does a lot of throat clearing and coughs raucously into her hand. She spends time finding a note to begin the song, and asks everyone to begin on the count of four. And so it starts. But Edna-eski sings so passionately and so badly that no one can stay with the song for very long. The shock of her terrible singing gives way to much laughter, but Edna-eski perseveres, repeating the song.

> You are my sunshine, my only sunshine
> You make me happy, when skies are grey
> You'll never know dear, how much I love you
> Please don't take my sunshine away.

It is a remarkable thing that when Edna-eski retains her enthusiasm and passion, people rise to meet her at that level of performance. They yell out the chorus and lift their arms and heads and point to each other for 'you' on the line 'I love you.' It is utter joy!

Benefits of singing

Singing lifts the spirit and reduces stress. Every community and care home should have a singing group; every domestic home needs a regular singsong! Qualitative studies show singing improves quality of life and well-being. It helps people breathe more deeply and take in more oxygen, which is good for the brain. Welch (2008) explains that singing creates links across multiple sites in the brain: visual, emotional, motor, sound and language processing (see also Barbershop Harmony Society 2010).

A study of community singing clubs in the UK by Skingley and Bungay (2010) found people reported feeling enjoyment; better mental health and well-being; increased social interaction; improvements in physical health; cognitive stimulation and learning; as well as improved memory and recall. The joyfulness was the most common response participants identified.

People enjoy learning new songs as well as the old familiars. There is a vast range of songs to choose from: African American spiritual songs; traditional folk; songs from the 1940s to 1960s; hymns; country songs; blues; pop; and songs of the homelands. Spend time finding out people's favourite songs and find the lyrics. Some care homes buy in or make several copies of song lyrics in large print for group sessions.

Singing can happen anywhere, whether solo, in pairs or groups. There is something fulfilling about singing with other people. Livesey *et al.* (2012) explored the benefits of choral singing. The social aspect was very important. People built networks and friendships. There was also an increased sense of purpose.

'Singing for the Brain': Alzheimer's Society

'Singing for the Brain' groups began in 2003 following a pilot study by Montgomery-Smith and Brennan (2003). The sessions are designed to improve confidence, self-esteem and quality of life for people with dementia and their carers. People are supported to sing, clap, hum, whistle and exercise in a friendly and social environment.

Carers and people with dementia, who might otherwise be feeling isolated at home, get the chance to socialise with people who share similar experiences. People usually chat over tea or coffee before the voice and body warm-up exercises.

Many groups begin with a 'welcome song', in which every member is named and greeted. This can be a beautiful and much appreciated ritual. Carers describe their partners 'coming alive' when the group sings their name. The rest of the songs usually incorporate hand or body movements. Action songs increase exercise and oxygen intake.

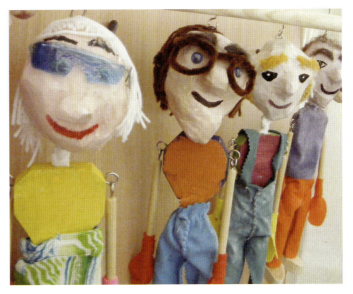

'The wise ones' – puppets of and by people with dementia

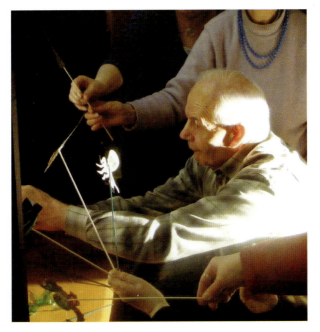

Dick and his peers perform someone's story with shadow puppets

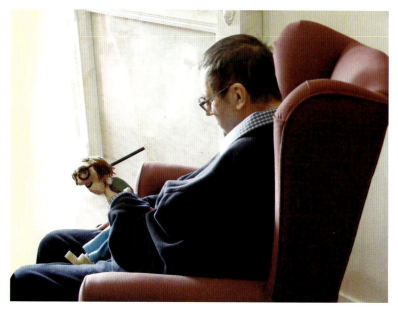

Jimpy contemplates, while his puppet peers around the room

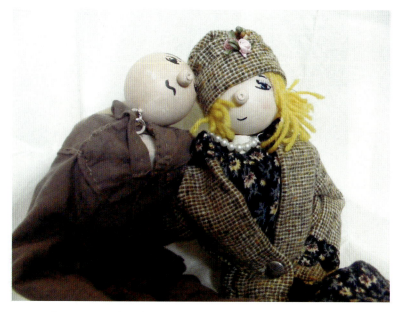

The war couple. A love story told by someone with dementia

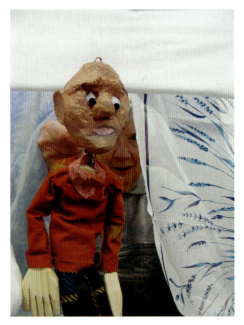

Mr Hasting's soul-puppet performance

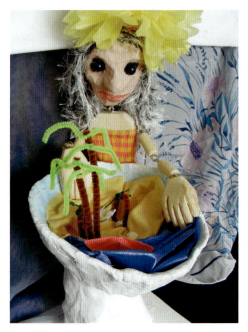

A family carer's dream of a two-week holiday

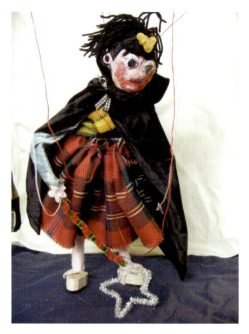

'Me as a fairy godmother' by participant of a mental health project

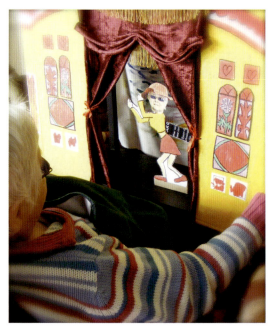

June and her model cartoon theatre puppet

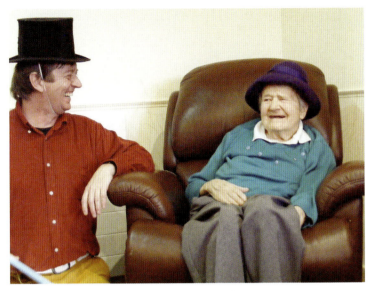

'I'm getting married in the morning'

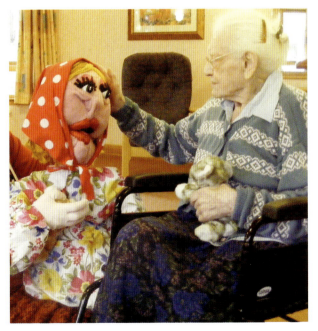

Margaret hums to the puppet whilst holding her kitten

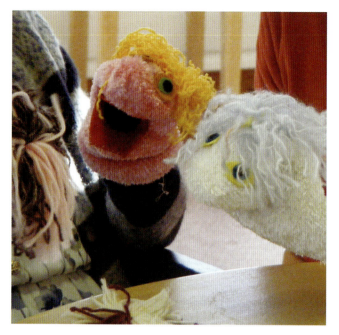

Singing sock puppets group activity

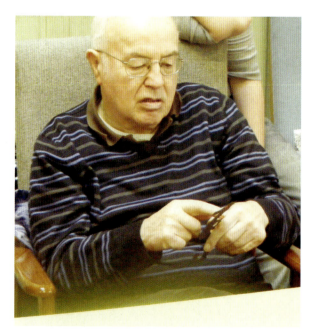

Murdo studies the shadow puppet he made

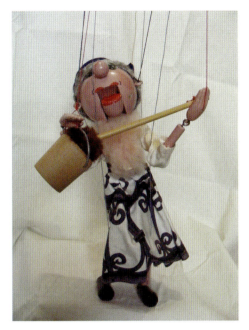

A Pelham Puppet – old lady with mop and bucket

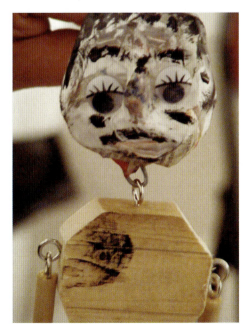

'Me as a Fisherman' rod puppet by participant of a mental health project

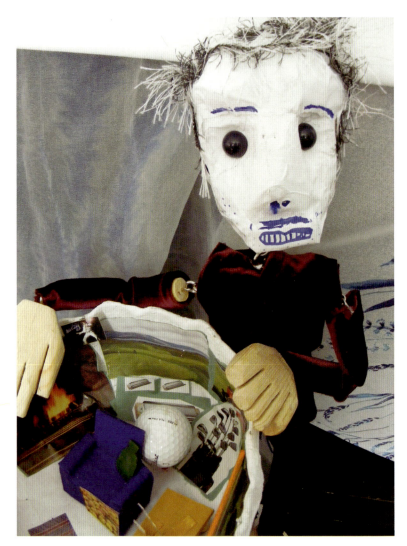

'He's had a shock, but he can still sing like Elvis.'
Participant with vascular dementia explains he wants home comforts

Do it yourself

If there is not a singing club nearby, you could set one up. You may just want to run things informally to begin with. But there are many established singing clubs (not just for people with dementia) who can pass on useful tips. Warm-ups are important and help to avoid voice strain, as well as establishing good breathing patterns. The vocal exercises help people feel more confident about singing.

The BBC (2013) has a variety of 'learn to sing' online videos with warm-ups and singing tips. You can also find singing warm-up ideas designed for older people online. People might prefer to start with a facial warm-up – gentle massaging, tapping, stretching, yawning, and generally pulling strange faces. Breathing exercises help centre and prepare people. Individuals may enjoy doing a general all-over body wake-up routine, or exercises at intervals through the session. Some people tend to slouch or fold in on themselves, so exercise and singing can help open the chest to breathe more deeply.

Gentle humming at various pitches works well for creating initial vocal sounds. People can feel the vibration of humming. Take time in the beginning so people can experience the resonance between themselves at different pitches. Moving from humming into all the vowel sounds gets the mouth and chords working.

To stay in tune, it can be useful to have an instrument such as a woodwind recorder to establish what the first note is for each song. You could record the beginning of each song on your mobile phone, as a reminder for the note to start with.

For singing at home, use CDs to sing along to if it feels easier to have accompaniment. There are karaoke channels on the Internet, which highlight the words to sing, while providing the backing tracks. If you enjoy hymns, there are religious services on the radio and television, as well as live stream from some churches through the Internet.

Some people fear they will be out of tune or have been told they sing badly. One man was told never to sing again by a schoolmaster. It took most of his life to find out how much he loved singing. Singing through a puppet is one way to overcome embarrassment, which is how Edna-eski got started on her singing career.

Songs, music and memory

Singing together has a feeling of camaraderie, equality and cooperation. Group singing allows for more dimensions to the songs, such as singing in rounds, or harmonies, male and female parts or one song over another. I have often sung with people who may barely have spoken in months, or their sentences were fragmented. But the song tunes and lyrics are remembered. How and why this happens is the subject of many research papers.

The brain seems able to connect creatively, as witnessed in our work. Rhyme, rhythm and the repetitive nature of songs are strong factors for remembering. The mental imagery that songs inspire also helps. What we do know is that music and songs have emotional impact.

Schulkind, Hennis and Rubin (1999) found that emotion had a significant effect on older people's memories of a song (the title, lyrics, recording artist) above and beyond any effect of familiarity of the song. It was not clear whether the memories create the emotion or the emotion brings out the memory. But music, emotion and memory of the song seem closely linked.

Earlier studies by Rubin (1995) show the importance of music for transmitting cultural information through ballads (songs that tell stories). The storing and retelling of ballads has happened over many generations, so perhaps the brain has developed greater ability to recall songs than other memories.

More recent research suggests the music and songs are stored in a different part of the brain from the hippocampus (seahorse-shaped parts of the limbic system). Finke, Esfahani and Ploner (2012) studied a man who had lost most of his memory, due to temporal lobe damage. He could neither recall his past, nor plan for his future. However, he could still play the cello and he learned new pieces of music.

Studies of people with amnesia by Haslam and Cook (2002, p.465) also show that people have an ability to learn and remember songs, even though other memories are not retrieved. This is thought to be due to the strength of the music. Without melody, the lyrics are less likely to be remembered.

In their review of ways in which music and singing relate to health and well-being, Stacy, Brittain and Kerr (2002) affirm that music can induce relaxation and have physical, emotional, spiritual and social benefits. They also highlight that music is an integral part of many cultures:

Music may accompany every activity from the cradle to the grave, through lullabies, games and dances, work songs, battle music, and at ceremonies and rituals, including those for life events such as coming of age, weddings and funerals. (Gregory 1997, cited in Stary *et al.* 2002, p.156)

Music scribbles

Music has the power to inspire and uplift us. A favourite creative activity of mine is to have a large sheet of paper and colour felt pens or crayons to do music scribbles. A piece of classical music is played loudly, such as 'Ode to Joy' from Beethoven's Symphony no. 9, Strauss's 'The Blue Danube' or Mozart's 'Eine Kleine Nachtmusik' (Allegro). The only rule is to let the felt pen or crayons dance across the page in response to the music.

This can be done individually or in small groups. It is interesting to look at the results and compare responses to the music. Sometimes it is possible to pick out the marks belonging to particular parts of the tune. Some music-dance-scribbles are beautiful pieces of art in their own right, with great swirls from the sound of sweeping violins, or tiny squiggles of staccato notes. People may use different colours to represent different aspects of the music, or a fistful of colours at the same time. I like to play the music a second time as this allows time for people to feel their way into the activity.

Singing socks

Singing sock puppets are easy to make, comical, sweet and perfectly suited to singing (see appendices). Most people find it easy to put their hand inside the sock to create a large mouth. The thumb fits in the heel and forms the bottom jaw. The rest of their fingers form the top of the jaw in the toe part of the sock, and the arm becomes the body of the being.

We usually put felt-covered card or plastic on the mouth, to stiffen the jaw, and hold its shape more definitely. The felt colour can be in contrast to the sock colour, which helps people see each other's puppet mouths. When the jaw is closed, the contrasting colour cannot be seen. This makes open mouths more obvious. In mid and later stages of dementia, people need every clue to make the tasks achievable.

Occasionally someone will need help to get his or her hand in the right position, and support to open and close the mouth.

Physical factors, such as arthritis, or cognitive issues affecting the person's ability to know which way up their hand is, can be overcome with gentle guiding. The exercise becomes more fun when attempting to synchronise hand movements to lyrics.

The thumb and fingers part to open the sock puppet mouth and emphasise certain words. Small movements with the finger and thumb nearer together convey the words in between. A song that could work well in this fashion by emphasising the 'oh' sound is 'There's No Business Like Show Business' written by Irving Berlin in 1946 (Rodgers and Hammerstein copyright and Universal Music Publishing Group for lyrics).

With practice, the synchronisation becomes very professional looking. Having words to emphasise helps to retain a steady rhythm. There is a tendency, noticed also by Dowling (1995, p.106), for people with dementia to speed up when they are singing. People sometimes sing right through the places where there should be gaps in a song. Playing an instrument or clapping a beat can work well to hold the tempo.

Singing sock puppets can be made to look like a church choir, with little white collars and black material on the body. This means people need to lift their forearms up a little higher to get the full effect. More movement can be added, such as swaying the arm, which opens the body of the puppeteer for better breathing. Swap arms so both sides are exercised. Hymns and Christmas carols will never be the same after singing sock puppets.

People may enjoy creating new lyrics or adding unique lines to familiar songs. One quiet man joined a group sock singing session. There was quite a gathering including family members and care home staff. During a pause between the verse and the chorus the man delivered a humorous line that made everyone laugh. He was thrilled with the response and became more energised.

Following the song the man chatted to us. We soon realised he was using words from lyrics of other songs although it sounded like ordinary speech at first. This prompted us to reply in song lyrics, which led to further singing. This was a valuable opportunity for the gentleman to lead the group.

It is important to try different songs and find out what people enjoy. During a creative learning programme for care staff, our singing puppets (Maggie and Rocky) visit people confined to bed with a few song books. Many staff already sing, and find the sessions affirmative. Singing is empowering for everyone involved and highly recommended.

Warning

Before printing and distributing lyrics from the Internet, read them first! I was running late for an evening singing group and had not prepared any new songs. We had enjoyed singing harmonies with traditional and Bluegrass-style songs, so I searched online for more and found 'My Grandfather's Clock' (written in 1876 by Henry C. Work).

> My grandfather's clock
> Was too large for the shelf,
> So it stood ninety years on the floor;
> It was taller by half
> Than the old man himself,
> Though it weighed not a pennyweight more.
> It was bought on the morn
> Of the day that he was born,
> It was always his treasure and pride;
> But it stopped short
> Never to go again,
> When the old man died.
> Ninety years without slumbering,
> Tick, tock, tick, tock,
> His life seconds numbering,
> Tick, tock, tick, tock,
> It stopped short
> Never to go again,
> When the old man died.

I printed the lyrics and rushed off to the session. A new person joined us that evening. It was exciting to hear she had received classical singing training, although our group was not in that league. In fact it became even further removed from anything classical when I handed out the lyrics. There was a shocked silence and then some giggling, but generally a sense of disturbance as the words were not as they should have been. The word 'clock' was missing the second letter and the whole song was about how it was too big for his pants, and dragged on the floor, but remained his pride and joy. The new person did not return.

CHAPTER 9

The Dying Lady with a Diva on Her Bed

The World of Bed Theatre

Fran seems to be disengaged from everything around her. Her eyes stare into space, as though looking beyond the ceiling. Her carers are concerned about her. She seems so unhappy, but she is not connecting. Everyone senses she has given up on life, and is simply waiting to pass away.

I sit in her room for a short while. Fran does not acknowledge me, just continues staring at the corner of the ceiling; sometimes panting; occasionally silent tears rolling down her cheeks. I hold her hand. She is in a white room. There are white walls, white ceiling, pale curtains and white bed linen.

On the next occasion, I gently float a red scarf into the space her eyes stare into. After a few billowing and fluttering movements, Fran's eyes flicker. She seems to focus. On subsequent occasions two people stand either side of Fran's bed and float various scarves up to her ceiling. We begin to make them dance above her duvet, and she watches. One day Fran smiles and nods.

One week it feels utterly inappropriate to do anything creative or colourful; such is the level of her despair. We just sit with Fran and cry with her. Not in a dramatic way, just a beingness that feels the desolateness. It is one of the few times Fran looks at me.

The next time I see Fran, she mouths 'thank you'. She clearly remembers the connection from a week before. Her eyes follow the scarves down from the ceiling and there is a dramatic-looking Diva puppet, in a tight red dress and sparkly shoes, dancing at the end of Fran's bed. Fran's face is a picture of surprise.

It may seem counter-intuitive to have such a lively puppet visiting someone so very frail and dying, but Fran seems to love the puppet. It would be more difficult for a human to take this initiative in case it was in poor taste, but a puppet can get away with it! The puppet can lead the way. There is a fine balance that carers and artists must strike, between being respectful of the peace and tranquillity for end of life care, and being respectful of the creative life energy still flowing.

The three-quarters human size Diva stands on the bed. She leans back as she does a high kick. Fran, whose face is often contorted with pain, bursts out laughing. The Diva blows her kisses as she does the splits. Fran keeps on laughing. For these few minutes she seems utterly transformed and free.

This level of interaction gives permission for staff to be 'bigger' around Fran. They had become so quiet around her. This is partly because communication is so difficult, and partly a perception that being silent is appropriate care when a person is dying. Now staff can be more present, more lively and comical, with 'ta-dahs' or songs when they enter her room. It does not stop Fran from dying, but it brings some joyfulness and relieves her (even momentarily) from pain.

Palliative care

People comment on the lovely and lively atmosphere of hospice settings. End of life care can be life affirming, with a deep compassion for the person. Life is celebrated and appreciated. There is a respect for the individual and a sense of offering the best, so the remaining time is used well. Palliative care offers support for people to live as actively as possible, and to adjust to their illness or disease, living well until death.

It has often struck me as strange that these principles are applied less when a person has years to live (or when a person has limited communication due to cognitive decline). A person should not have to be dying before he or she receives compassionate care that celebrates life. In order to have this more uplifting attitude to care, family carers and care staff need to feel more supported. In care settings regular and effective supervision helps staff to identify best practice. Family carers could benefit from similar opportunities to discuss ethical, emotional and practical care issues.

End of life care aims to promote quality of life, through comfort and pain relief, dignity and support. Carers help relieve stress. They support individuals dealing with fears about death and dying. Mares (2003, pp.74–77) highlights the importance of offering opportunities for people to talk about their fears. These include fear of pain; of ceasing to exist; of losing control; of being buried alive; of being a burden; of being separated from the loved ones; and of dying alone. Some people fear they cannot make amends or resolve long-standing issues. Palliative work can bring great comfort and peace.

When a person is dying of brain disease affecting communication, we may not know if these fears are present. If no plans or discussion are established earlier in life, it may be helpful to address the issues in terms of what can be done. For example, explain that if the person shows signs of pain, the doctor can offer pain relief. Offer to arrange visits from a person of faith or to read passages from books of comfort. Set intentions to create moments of wonder or connection.

Palliative care includes helping people clarify how they want to spend their time, and what types of treatment they want. Few people with dementia die in a hospice setting. The European World Health Organization palliative care report explains that this type of care was originally developed for people with cancer (Davies and Higginson 2004). The service was extended to people with similar needs (e.g. people with heart disease).

There have been years of debate about whether dementia is a terminal illness. Death certificates are found to be unreliable because people with dementia often die of other illnesses, so the dementia is not recorded as the direct cause of death (World Health Organization and Alzheimer's Disease International 2012, p.56).

The prognosis for people diagnosed with dementia is individual and variable. It depends at what stage the illness is diagnosed, age of the person being diagnosed, the environment, level of fitness, rates of progression and whether the person has other illnesses, such as heart disease, pulmonary disease or diabetes. Death from these diseases means the person dies with dementia rather than of it. Many people in later stages of dementia die of pneumonia (Van Der Steen *et al.* 2009, p.141).

There is growing recognition that the advanced stages of dementia are terminal. Even though the different forms of dementia have different patterns of progress, the severe stages of each have the same symptoms and clinical problems regardless of the initial diagnosis (Volicer 2010).

There are different 'scales' describing stages of dementia, which can help people get an overall sense of the pattern of the diseases, but as stated all through this book, the journey is personal. Reisberg *et al.* (1982) developed a scale that measures decline in cognitive function – the Global Deterioration Scale (GDS) for Assessment of Primary Degenerative Dementia. Two years later Reisberg developed the more popular scale based on the level of functioning on daily activities, such as the ability to dress or feed oneself. This scale is called the Functional Assessment Staging Tool (FAST) (Reisberg 1984, cited in Reisberg and Sclan 1992, pp.58–59).

Stages 1 and 2 are normal ageing functions. The early period of dementia can be matched to stages 3 and 4, where there is a more noticeable memory loss or difficulty with financial transactions and organising. People may live with dementia for many years without other people realising the person is living with brain disease.

The middle phase of dementia is associated with stages 5 and 6. There is a more noticeable change, and a gradual increase in help required for daily living tasks. People could need help with what to wear or what to eat. This may progress to how to get dressed and how to eat. The mid to late phase (stage 6) may also include incontinence and inability to bathe properly. These first six stages may last for several years. Not every person has every symptom.

Stage 7 is the late or severe phase of dementia when the person is unable to communicate verbally, or walk without assistance and is completely dependent for all daily living needs. It seems that dying is not mentioned very much in policies about dementia care (Kellehear 2009), although this later stage is regarded as terminal. According to Dooneief *et al.* (1996), the average survival rate in this late stage is one year. However, we are now used to the fact that cancer and Aids prognoses are more variable than the given timescales, so it is important to remain open.

People with advanced dementia should have the same respect and consideration afforded to people living and dying with other terminal illnesses. It is a time when people are at their most vulnerable. When carers feel there is nothing to be done except attend to basic needs, the person they are caring for is likely to be in the later stages of dementia. Remember there are ways to connect beyond words, as we saw in Chapter 4, and people still appreciate feelings of love and joy.

What really matters is having the best quality of life possible at any point in life, with or without dementia. When people become confined to bed, they continue to have needs and desires that carers can help fulfil. Living in one room, or one environment day after day, can be mind-numbing. While quiet times and rest times are needed, people really appreciate sparks of life and connection. Boredom causes apathy and apathy can lead to depression. Fresh flowers, a new picture, and a change of curtains – these can help lift the spirits.

Gentle physical care can make a huge difference. Brush or comb hair; gently massage the face or hands. Help the person keep their mouth clean and moist. Mouth hygiene is an area often neglected in people who have become dependent. According to De Oliveira (2010, p.3) poor oral hygiene increases the risk of cardiovascular disease. Reduced toothbrushing is associated with higher levels of C-reactive protein and fibrinogen, which are present when inflammation occurs. This highlights the importance of good oral hygiene. Although I have not yet seen a definitive link between oral hygiene and dementia, I am interested in the reviews by Kuo *et al.* (2005) that conclude that C-reactive protein is linked to stroke and cognitive disorders. Carers can do no harm in promoting mouth hygiene.

Psychologically carers can do much to lighten people's experience of being bed-bound. We can make rooms more beautiful, comfortable and interesting. Creative thinking helps carers to break the monotony of the same walls and decor. One lady loved having her bed covered in different coloured materials. A gentleman enjoyed seeing old postcards of steam trains tacked to his ceiling. Balloons and fairy lights help celebrate any anniversary.

If short of materials, use a bed sheet to create a puppet in the style of the scarf puppet in Chapter 2. The sheet puppet with its huge knot-head and knot-hand could explore the room, looking and pointing at the most ordinary of things. The naivety of the puppet instils a sense of wonder in the audience member. One gentleman seemed in awe as he watched the puppet look at the lampshade, inside and out, and examine items on his trolley. The bed-sheet puppet was a regular source of entertainment with him.

Duvet, sheets and blankets can create the most wonderful landscapes, as depicted in 'The Land of Counterpane' by Robert Louis Stevenson (1973).

> When I was sick and lay a-bed,
> I had two pillows at my head,
> And all my toys beside me lay,
> To keep me happy all the day.
>
> And sometimes for an hour or so
> I watched my leaden soldiers go,
> With different uniforms and drills,
> Among the bed-clothes, through the hills;
>
> And sometimes sent my ships in fleets
> All up and down among the sheets;
> Or brought my trees and houses out,
> And planted cities all about.
>
> I was the giant great and still
> That sits upon the pillow-hill,
> And sees before him, dale and plain,
> The pleasant land of counterpane.

Esther has spent over a year in bed. English is not her first language, and she rarely speaks. The staff play music from her culture and help her eat and drink. They make her as comfortable as possible. Her carers gradually find there are more creative things they can do to connect with Esther.

We use soft wool to play a version of 'cat's cradle'. This is a hand game that uses string or wool to create different patterns, known in different forms around the world. The game can become complicated, so we begin with unravelling and wrapping wool. During one session, Esther's hand feels along the wool, and comes to my hand. She wraps a piece of wool, then feels my hand further and clasps her hand in mine.

We make patterns on Esther's bed with the long strands of wool. One day we introduce a basket of wool with a puppet kitten inside it. Esther's eyes light up, and more puppet kittens arrive. Kittens are often associated with playing with balls of wool, so this is an everyday kind of narrative that Esther seems to understand.

Our new version of cat's cradle is a kinaesthetic joke on our earlier attempts. The kittens pull the wool into all sorts of patterns above Esther's bed. We are all entangled in the wool, and Esther laughs as we try to untangle the big mess.

This progression builds over several ten-minute sessions. Sometimes we sing or hum tunes as we work. Esther focuses for longer periods and one day makes kitten 'meow' sounds, when the puppets arrive. The sessions become more elaborate dancing with wool and kittens over and above her bed. Esther's knees make great hills for the kittens to slide down. A giant bird arrives, and Esther makes the clucking sounds of a hen. These sessions are always brief because Esther tires easily. But each week the connection grows, which encourages her carers to stay and chat a while or sing a song.

The interactions help everyone involved. It is important not to force an interaction or activity; but the opportunities and offers should be regularly available. Beds can become changing depictions of life stories. Handwritten cards can record life events, achievements, favourite people and places. These can be pegged or taped onto the bedcover. Ribbons link up the life events. The activity feels more participative than showing someone a photo-album, but each way of connecting is valuable if the person enjoys it.

The small theatre being made in Chapter 6 is lightweight enough to be used on beds and wheelchairs. Model theatre ideas are excellent for being performed at the bedside. Create one to sit on the bedside table, and make model cartoon puppets depicting the family members or carers and friends. I have found this to be more fun than using the traditional models.

However, the traditional model theatre does have its place, and there is something both beautiful and satisfying about making a well-known show together. The story of Cinderella (published by Charles Perrault over 300 years ago) has recognisable elements of life, and an outcome that offers comfort. The main character faces struggles, hardships, uncertainty, hope, fortunate interventions and eventual success. Creating the show involves colouring in and cutting out. It is, as Robert Louis Stevenson (1895) enthused, a delightful way to spend time. The Victoria and Albert Museum (2013) in London offers a Cinderella kit to print off and make.

A person confined to bed can also be involved in making their own hand puppets and rod puppets, or performing short pieces of narrative and script. In later stages of dementia, the bedside theatre work is often a form of participatory theatre as with the cat's cradle described above. It is important to build the activities a little at a time, and ensure the person is happy to continue.

Our singing puppets Maggie and Rocky meet people confined to bed who may be too frail to engage with some of the practical activities. When singing songs from musicals – for example 'My Favourite Things' from *The Sound of Music* – it is beautiful to hear the voice of someone who has not spoken, gaining strength through the familiar song. The imagery of raindrops on roses and whiskers on kittens, or brown paper packages tied up with string, is inspiring. Some men prefer love songs such as 'Maria' from *West Side Story* or 'Some Enchanted Evening' from *South Pacific*. It is as important for carers as it is for people dying of dementia or other long-term condition, to have these moments of light relief. Although dying is a serious issue, there is room for comedy, colour and creativity.

Advanced directives

A subject regularly explored in my work is about wishes and dreams. What do people really want in life? And what can we do as carers or family members or friends to help? It seems important that each of us clarifies what is important while we have cognitive abilities. We see many people who can no longer communicate their desires, and who have no statements about what they want in terms of treatment or care. This can cause great difficulty for family members who have their own values and beliefs and thoughts about what is best. We need to look at how death and dying can be better supported for everyone.

A report by the World Health Organization European Office shows that most studies find that 75 per cent of the general population would prefer to die at home (Davies and Higginson 2004, pp.16–17). In the United States, between 18 and 32 per cent do so. In the UK, around 21 per cent of people do so (Office for National Statistics 2011). Most deaths occur in nursing homes and hospitals. According to an Alzheimer's Society report (Kane 2012, p.34), only 6 per cent of people with dementia as the cause on the death certificate died at home; 63 per cent died in a care home and 30 per cent died in hospital.

We need to get better at meeting people's needs. Better at having discussions about death and dying, and palliative care. We do not have to have a diagnosis or a terminal illness to write down what our preferences are for future care. Consider what you would like to be continued if your support needs became high due to an accident or serious disease. What are your values? What would be a perfect day? What is non-negotiable? Where would you want to die if possible? What sort of burial service would you like? Make a note of these things and let someone know the information exists.

An advanced directive or living will is a statement about what sort of medical treatment you would rather not have if you ever reached a point of lacking mental capacity. These discussions need to happen early on in the diagnosis of dementia, or even without a diagnosis, even though there may be several years of living well. The document can be changed to suit changing needs, but can only be done while the person is deemed to have mental capacity to make such decisions.

Having mental capacity means having the ability to understand and retain information, and to make a choice based on that information. Having dementia does not mean the person lacks mental capacity; they may just need longer to communicate or the language rephrased.

There are mental competence or capacity laws throughout the world. The UK Mental Capacity Act 2005 assumes that every adult has mental capacity (unless proven otherwise) and that each person has the right to make decisions.[1] The Act also upholds the right for individuals to make eccentric or unwise decisions. (This is excellent news for people who enjoy dangerous sports!)

An advanced directive may be something along the following statement: 'If I only have a few weeks to live and am unable to communicate and have irreversible brain damage, or am in a coma, and unlikely to regain consciousness, then the treatment I want is for relieving pain and not treatment to prolong the dying.'

But things may not be so clear and direct. It is worth discussing various outcomes. For example, I currently think I would like to stay alive if I was aware, even if I could not guarantee making myself understood. Being totally dependent on others feels very scary, but many people do it and I have met many kind and compassionate carers. I have also met people who exchanged joyfulness, love, wisdom and kindness in situations that sometimes seemed hopeless. One lady in her mid nineties had been dying in her bed for a few weeks. One morning she seemed remarkably energised and lucid. She was keen to be up and dressed.

Her husband and son were utterly amazed, for they were preparing for her death. In the kitchen the lady wanted to make banana sandwiches and go for a picnic on this summer day. Her son said he would drive us around the beautiful Highland roads. The lady and I sat in the back with blankets. We stopped briefly beside a river to eat our banana sandwiches, with the sun reflected in the water.

Just as we returned to the car, a golden eagle flew ahead of us. Such a huge wingspan and a mighty bird that we watched it for a while as it headed further west. Everybody was thrilled. It was a special day. When the lady returned to her bed she did not get up again, but her husband spoke with her about seeing the golden eagle. That day has stayed with me for over 15 years as a reminder to never assume someone's life is over until he or she decides it is.

All around the world, people with mental capacity can give someone the authority to make decisions about their financial affairs and health and welfare matters. Some people ask their family members to have the power of attorney, others ask friends. These lasting or enduring powers of attorney are legally binding, but can be changed while the person has mental capacity.

Any decisions taken on behalf of another person who does not have capacity must be made in their best interests, and have the least restrictive impact on the person's freedom. Written statements help people make the right decisions, and ensure that care and treatment is as person-centred as possible.

Recent chats with people with dementia and people with experiences of increasing memory loss or cognitive decline showed a variety of wishes: to visit places around the world; to find a new partner; to die at home with friends drinking champagne; to be free from arthritic pain; to find lost children; to hear certain audio books; to see grandchildren; to meet the Queen; to be on TV.

When children are receiving end of life care, we do our best to fulfil their wishes. We recognise the importance of helping children feel as fulfilled as possible. The Make-A-Wish Foundation is an international organisation created for this purpose. For adults, the US Dream Foundation works with over 600 hospices and healthcare organisations to fulfil dreams, provide peace, closure and joy for adults at the end of their lives.[2] There are international organisations linked to hospices helping adults achieve their dying wishes. This work can be extended to include people with dementia. Carers become increasingly aware that as communication and cognitive function deteriorates individual wishes and dreams are not so easily recognised.

So we must work intuitively and creatively – remembering the journey goes beyond alienation into wonderment. People in the very late stages of dementia are in transition between life and death. We can connect through music, song, puppetry, colour, poetry, drama, love and joy.

Notes

1. For the Mental Capacity Act 2005, see www.legislation.gov.uk/ukpga/2005/9/contents. For the code of practice in Scotland, Adults with Incapacity (Scotland) Act 2000: Code of Practice, see www.scotland.gov.uk/Publications/2008/03/20114619/0.

2. For Make-A-Wish International, see http://worldwish.org. For Make-A-Wish UK, see www.make-a-wish.org.uk. For the US Dream Foundation, see www.dreamfoundation.org.

CHAPTER 10

Get Me that Red Lipstick, I'm Going to the Ball

Self-Esteem through Puppetry

Gerty lifts her head off the pillow when Rocky puppet arrives. Sometimes Gerty is irritated with her visitors, but never with Rocky. In recent weeks she has been talking about Rocky to the carers between visits. Rocky with his proud ways matches Gerty's big personality. They hold hands and he tells her what a fine looking lady she is, and she asks him what his job is as he is wearing such a good suit. The puppet considers the question, but Gerty has already decided he is a news reporter, and she has some stories for him.

This time the narrative is about stolen things: teeth, necklace, house and purse. In metaphorical world, these things all link to loss of independence and identity. Gerty is becoming upset as she lists her injuries. Rocky replies in his usual big and affirmative way:

> *'Is that so! Well, that sounds really hard. I'm so glad you are here all safe and sound, Gerty.'*

And she squeezes his hand and notices Rocky is wearing a rose in his jacket pocket. She wonders if he is off to a wedding, but he replies, no, the rose is for her. Gerty grins from ear to ear! She tells Rocky he has made her day, her week, her year!

On another occasion, Gerty seems thrilled to meet the Diva puppet. The Diva has huge red lips and big eyes with blue feather eyelashes. Gerty looks the Diva up and down, and takes her hand. She touches the red dress, then notices the Diva has a necklace.

'That's the key,' she exclaims.

But she does not elaborate. Instead she talks as though narrating passing scenes. There are words about waiting for her daughter to get the bread; cleaning the house; the school gates; a letter for the bank; the dentist. Gerty pats the Diva's hand, then she stares for ages at the puppet's mouth.

'I want lipstick…deep rouge! … Get me that red lipstick!'

The following session we bring the lipstick and the Diva. While I put the lipstick on Gerty, she holds the Diva's hand and says they are going to the ball. Gerty suits the deep red lipstick and a sparkling red hat. She finds it hard to lift her head off the pillow, so I ask her if she would like to see herself in a handheld mirror. Gerty nods.

It is important to use mirrors with sensitivity. Some people may feel upset that they look older than they thought they were, or they may not recognise the reflection at all. Gerty spends almost twenty minutes looking at herself, as I hold the mirror above her. She touches her face and moves her head from side to side, keeping her eyes steady. Gerty's eyes are beautiful. I tell her I love seeing the colours in people's eyes. She looks deep into her eyes and says,

'Windows to the soul.'

After a while she fills her cheeks with air. She lets the air out and tries lifting her sagging cheeks. She smiles and says that nothing can stop it (ageing?). We sit in silence, and take turns holding the mirror as steady as possible, watching her movements. There are flickers of smile or furrows of frown. She tries different facial movements; some are very comical and we burst out laughing and spend a few minutes just pulling funny faces.

Other expressions are more serious. Then there is a deepening more meditative look, as she studies her own eyes again. The room feels very peaceful and full of gratitude. It is quite an extraordinary experience and a privilege to see someone connecting with who they are. For her remaining weeks, Gerty's carers continue using puppetry. Her love and humour ever near as she chats about who she is, and who the puppets are.

Identity

'Who am I?' is one of life's big questions, and the old theories still hold significance. Our identity is linked to our self-concept, and this begins in childhood. The child learns who he or she is by the way others respond, and by discovering what he or she likes. Rogers (1959) believed that people pick up messages about how acceptable or unacceptable they are in the early years, and then continue the pattern. For example, a child who is given positive feedback and appreciation is more likely to have higher self-esteem, and so feel worthy and able to achieve things.

Growing up with frequent criticism or being treated as inferior creates a negative self-image and lower self-esteem that can get in the way of achieving full potential. This condition can, however, change through conscious self-development work, and through favourable environments that nurture the person.

Roger's (1959) theory suggests that suffering occurs when there is a gap between how a person views himself or herself, and how they would really like to be. The narrower the gap, the more in harmony the person feels. Having a sense of integrity creates a positive outlook. If a person feels undervalued, he or she may struggle to find self-value. The person is more likely to have a more negative outlook on life.

The word 'identify' is derived from Latin 'idem', meaning 'the same'. This is interesting as we so often use the word identity to talk about what makes an individual uniquely different – not the same. Gerty identifies with the glamour of the Diva. She also seems clear about having her own identity, and it is important we help her maintain that sense of self. Other people we work with seem less concerned about identity. However, it is a subject carers think a lot about.

Erikson (1968) developed a theory about identity that took into account the influence of parents and society on the development of personality. He explained various stages that occur over a lifetime that everyone experiences from infancy to old age.

Each stage potentially strengthens individual identity, builds trust, self-reliance, purpose and competence. The identity is established in adolescence and the individual grows through intimacy and relationships. Healthy progress sees people wanting to create a better place for the next generation, and gaining integrity or wisdom. When a person feels confident and competent, they grow from strength to strength.

However, at each of these stages there are factors that can cause the person to experience negatives, such as mistrust, shame, guilt, inferiority, isolation and despair. These all lead away from feeling confident. During such experiences people may have an identity crisis. This is a state of confusion and anguish over what to do, or how to be. A person may behave differently. For example, he or she may suddenly withdraw or appear anxious and negative about life.

Identity crisis can happen at any time of significant transition in life. Losing a role causes major changes. It can take a long time to adjust to not being a partner or a full-time parent, or being out of employment. A change in one area of life has an influence on every other area. The person may feel unsure about everything they previously valued. It can be a painful time, and people benefit from empathetic support. Identity crisis can also be a time of fresh potential. Individuals discover new directions or reaffirm their life purpose.

For people with dementia, an identity crisis may be caused in the same way as for anyone else. It may also come about due to memory loss or inability to make sense of things that used to make sense. In the map shown in Figure 2 (see Chapter 3), a person experiencing identity crisis may be in the place before 'letting go', feeling confused and lost. Sometimes 'surrendering' to the experience, rather than fighting it, allows for a sense of relief. But it can be difficult to express what is happening.

One lady holds a puppet of herself close to her chest. At first I think she is regarding it as a baby or a doll. But she tells me it is her little self listening to her big self. When I ask what she can hear, she smiles and says she hopes it will tell her who she is. There has been no indication through the making process that this lady is struggling with her identity. She appears more confident than other people in crisis, but there is a gap for her that she wants to bridge.

Her puppet sits on her dressing table for days, but every now and then she holds it to her heart. One day I ask her if it is helping her know who she is, and she says,

> 'No, dear, but we're getting along quite well.'

It reminds me of a Russian fairy tale I know very well called Vasalisa. A dying mother gives her daughter, called Vasalisa, a doll that will always guide her to do the right thing at the right time in the right way. The doll represents the mother's intuition and it helps Vasalisa deal with many difficulties including the scary witch Baba Yaga – the one who knows. The witch knows a lot, but she cannot beat the mother's love and intuition held in the doll.

Even though the lady does not know who she is, she has a level of confidence that seems greater than any loss of identity. The puppet seems to offer some comfort. Losing identity is one of the biggest fears people have about dementia. Yet this may be more of an issue for the family members than the person diagnosed with dementia.

People diagnosed with early and mid stages of dementia are often keen to undertake life story work, with family members. The project may involve telling their story through words, imagery and creative process. I have been doing life story work for several years with people who use care services. People want to tell their story for a variety of reasons, from recording a memory so someone can remind them later, through to a burning desire to tell their version of events.

> There is no greater agony than bearing an untold story inside of you. (Angelou 2013)

Story work

Life story work can be as informal as chatting about different life themes, such as school days or special occasions. The work may be recorded as a way to help carers deliver person-centred care, or to understand more about a shared social history. The following points need to be considered:

- What would the life story work mean to the person telling it?
- Who would the information be shared with?
- Who would the person prefer not to share the information with?
- What happens if the person remembers things that are upsetting or distressing?
- What happens if the person changes his or her mind?
- Where will the story information be kept?
- Who does the story information belong to?

Life story work may cover the many areas we noted in Chapter 2 in addition to notes about the best times, comedy moments, dreams and wishes, support networks and so on. A life story can be presented as a book or booklet. Some people like to give these as gifts for close family members. Story photo-albums can be made using family photographs or relevant photos from magazines, with short written accounts of events. This can be made even more special with beautiful paper backgrounds and colourful motifs or ribbons throughout the book.

One relative made a stunning life story collage for his brother's house, which hangs on the living room wall, and helps visiting carers understand the bigger picture of family and place. The stories can be represented in cartoon form as comic strips, with exaggerated expressions showing important life moments. One man took up art in his late sixties to illustrate his life story book.

Another interesting representation is through the use of cloth. The material patterns might be from a particular era, or use favourite colours and textures. These can cover cardboard pages with material pockets or compartments for photos or written accounts, poems or postcards. The pages can be tied together with ribbon. Added features such as working buttons and zips sewn into the compartments give the story book a very personal and hands-on feel.

Non-literary stories can also be sewn into bed quilts or wall hangings using scraps of material. Or pieces cut from family members' clothes can be made into pictures describing the person's life events. The sewing of tapestries or quilts has long been used to depict social history and important cultural events. Working on such projects with or alongside the person with dementia offers a different way of connecting.

When someone's communication is not yet understood, and we do not know the person, it is important to maintain a sense of curiosity about him or her. Ask relatives and friends what they remember. However, we must realise these stories are about the relatives' and friends' views of the person, and not necessarily what the person would say about him or herself. Ultimately if the person is not telling his or her own story, the story is about someone else's experience. Continue to ask yourself questions such as the following:

Who is this person? What were they like as a child? What are their memories? What made them laugh? How did they cope with the tough times? Where have they felt safe or happy or scared? Who were their favourite people in the past? Whose voice or touch soothed them? Who read to them at night? What did they dream about? What funny incidents were they involved with? Where did they go on days out? What have they seen or heard? Who celebrated their achievements with them? What opportunities did they have to show their feelings? What concerts or parties did they enjoy? How do they feel about being here? What did they lose? What did they gain?

Keep open to the fact that each person has many stories whether or not they can tell us. Look for clues. Ask the person and listen with your ears and eyes. There are some questions we may not be able to know the answers to, but that does not mean they do not exist. There will be an answer, however hidden or secret, to every one of the above questions. Be aware of the whole person and their mysteries.

Making story or memory boxes is one of my favourite activities to do with people about their preferences. Shoeboxes can be decorated with fabric or magazine images, wrapping paper, or birthday cards chosen by the person (through pointing or noticing what the person looks at most). The objects and images placed in the box represent what people believe the person likes or dislikes. They are also reminders of places or shared activities that can generate 'conversation'.

If you go out together, notice what the person you are with seems interested in. Help them choose an object that represents your day out, such as an entrance ticket, a postcard, a pine cone from a walk, a shell, a feather, a label from a favourite food or drink, an ornament or model of an animal or boat or car. These physical objects can be placed in the person's 'story box' along with photographs and favourite song lyrics or CD covers.

The purpose of life story work varies depending on the level of interaction and engagement. For some people a life story helps maintain a sense of identity, connection and belonging. Relatives describe the experience as relaxing and therapeutic for themselves. Staff find the life story work interesting and helpful for conversations.

Puppets are perfect for people who want to tell their story 'anonymously'. The puppet screen or stage set provides a safe space for self-expression. This safe space can paradoxically be incredibly direct. Puppets are starkly uncompromising and unmistaken in their portrayal of a human story. Even the most simple of stories can take your breath away.

One participant portrayed a little puppet trying to untangle itself from various materials. It kept finding holes to peep through, but could not seem to get free. If it got close to escape, another swathe of material fell over it. The puppet struggle was set to music. There were no words for the story, and it was very powerful.

Sometimes we do not need to know what the story is. We enter a world with someone with puppets, and come out feeling something amazing just happened, but we do not have to know exactly what that is. There is a connection, and the connection is reached more quickly on subsequent visits.

Our work with people with dementia explores fragments or creates something in the moment. Some puppet stories are pure joy. Others are emotionally moving. Some stories do not have happy endings. The little puppet above never escapes the entanglement in that story. However, later, she is found poking her head out from the lady's handbag.

Making self puppets

We have seen that creative interactions and activities build self-esteem. People gain a sense of achievement. The very act of creating is highly stimulating and satisfying. Arts offer opportunities for people to be productive, and gain a sense of empowerment. Self-esteem increases our well-being and quality of life. In his article about the impact of arts on health, Cohen (2006b) explains that psycho-neuro-immunology (pni) scientists find positive feelings, associated with a sense of control, produce more T-cells that boost the immune system defences.

It is important the creative-making sessions offer opportunities to feel complete, and in control, even if the task is not finished. The person gains a sense of achievement, or at the very least experiences something of interest that they influence. Be clear about having a beginning and an end; even if the task is incomplete, you can still create an appreciative ending to the activity.

In the early and mid stages of dementia, people seem to value having a puppet of themselves. (I call it a self puppet or soul puppet.) Making this process accessible is a vital part of the work we do. It is important to think about each activity in advance of the session. Consider what is required: level of eyesight, dexterity, concentration and problem-solving. Sit with the person over a meal. This enables you to see whether a person is left or right handed, whether they can use cutlery, how strong their hands are, how far their arms can reach, their level of energy or interest. This knowledge helps tailor the creative activities to suit.

The wooden jointed puppets are more complex than hand puppets, but they are popular. It is relatively easy to prepare the wooden parts in advance (see appendices) so people get to do the sandpapering, painting and assembly themselves. Heads can be made using papier-mâché or wooden balls.

Papier-mâché has the benefit of being made into a head-shape that is a likeness to the individual's head. Some people enjoy the easy and physical making. We use torn-up newspaper and PVA glue, layered over a screwed up newspaper ball. Decide if the head is for a hand puppet, a rod puppet or a marionette at this stage. Each puppet form needs a different technical application to be incorporated into the making: wooden dowel for rod puppet, wire hoops for marionette or neck opening for the hand puppet (see appendices).

Often there is an immediate and spontaneous mini-performance with the puppet when it is complete. Other times we work with the individual to create something. We usually do this by focusing attention on the puppet, asking the puppet questions or wondering out loud whether the puppet can do certain things.

Bert becomes very talkative through his rod puppet. It is dressed in a fisherman's outfit and becomes more powerful each visit. He uses his puppet to tell everyone about the time he tossed the caber at the Highland games.

'It went over 200 yards … Aye… I won a silver medal for it.'

For a while, everyone basks in Bert's obvious glory. Creativity has no boundaries. No exclusion zones. Anything is possible. Bert and his puppet bring much joy. There is no greater recognition of the meaning and importance of a puppet when we heard a few months later that Bert's puppet attended his funeral.

We do not have to step in and make the happy ending. Our role is to honour the story, in whatever way it is told. It is enough to be with the person, and 'hold' the space with unconditional positive regard. The beauty of puppetry is the externalisation and expression of human experiences in all stages of life.

Mr J. does not use his puppet to tell any particular story. He recognises the puppet as himself when the nurse gives it to him. He checks its big glasses and touches his own. He looks at it and spends a long time touching the pieces he painted. He feels over the contours, and sits it on his lap. It is poignant to watch a man who struggles to see, sitting in a great armchair, with a little version of himself peering around the room.

One lady expresses her lifelong desire to be an artist as she slowly and meticulously paints part of the facade for another little puppet theatre. A few weeks later, Rocky the news reporter puppet visits the lady with a photograph of herself painting. He expresses his delight at meeting her:

'I hear you are a famous artists!' he declares.

The lady takes a few minutes to consider this encounter. She looks at the photograph, then leans back in her chair. Rocky puppet remains steady; the expectation for connection has already happened. For a while the lady holds her chin, in the classic thinker's pose. Eventually the lady leans forward, speaking to Rocky puppet:

'Yes, it's true.'

Validation and self-esteem

Validation of a person's experiences, feelings and values is another important aspect of dementia care. James (2008) highlights the importance of spotting the underlying sense or emotion the person is conveying, and giving a response to that. It is about accepting a person's reality and responding to that in a way that feels genuine and compassionate.

Gerty's increasing anxiety about things being stolen was validated when the general sense of loss was acknowledged, and her safety was affirmed. It is still important to record and report the allegations of theft, because such claims should never be overlooked. However, these things can be investigated and discussed further when Gerty is less upset. What matters is that she feels safe.

There was no need to correct Bert on the fact that tossing a caber is not about distance, or that 200 yards would be unlikely, because the main point is to validate his sense of pride, his wonderful imagination and his ability to share his joyfulness. Carers are better at understanding the importance of valuing individual feelings, and of creating positive interactions. Feelings matter. They influence individual well-being.

The carers need to find the place that is honest so they can respond to people with integrity and congruence. People with dementia are often more sensitive to body language and can tell if someone is not being honest.

> Validation teaches that we never lie to the person who has dementia because we need to establish their trust in order to validate their feelings. When we lie we lose their trust because on some level they already know the truth. (Feil 2012)

So we must find the place of truth, and that is invariably where the feelings are. When Ian searches for money to tip the waiter at dinnertime, some staff tell him he is in a care home. This distresses Ian, because he believes he is in a restaurant. It is important to validate how Ian feels. He feels good when he has a few coins in his pocket to leave on the table. He's a successful man about his business, and able to eat out. We can talk with him about his favourite restaurants and about his life as a businessman.

When Rose seems pleased that you are her mother, be glad that Rose feels a sense of safety or love in your presence. Breathe into the moment to gain clarity about what to say next. You do not have to say anything. You could simply hold her hand. Or you might ask what her favourite time was with her mum. Her feelings for her mum are validated. Later you might return to the room with a cheery 'Hi Rose, it's [real name] here.'

If Rose thinks you are the scum of the earth, and believes you cheated on her even before you were born, take some breaths to gather yourself. You might decide to change the subject to something bright and cheerful that diverts Rose off the subject. But if Rose is insistent about her claim, then you might acknowledge her feelings of anger and hurt more directly. The Rocky puppet could say with great enthusiasm:

'Gee Rose! What a terrible thing to happen to you! I like you very much. I hope we can be friends.'

If Mr D. is convinced you are stealing his cutlery, breathe first, while assessing what Mr D. is feeling. Does he regard himself as head of the household? In which case affirm his importance in the house, and your role in cleaning the cutlery, if that is what you do. Would he like to inspect the fine cutlery or other items around the house? He could draw up an itinerary of everything in the home, if at home. Or he could help with monthly audits in the care home. His advisers can deal with everything else so he can relax.

Self-identity and esteem are what person-centred approaches are all about. Carers promote the individuality and uniqueness of a being. However, the journey embarked to maintain individuality is rarely smooth. Other people's responses may be undermining. Sometimes the label of dementia creates a sense of limitation and a narrowing of choices. There are large misconceptions about people diagnosed with dementia, and if left unchallenged the stigma prevents progress.

Shifts in attitudes and understanding do happen, as we have witnessed with people with learning difficulties (intellectual disabilities). Less than 50 years ago, when people expressed hopes of independence, they were met with disbelief that this would be possible.

The human rights movement, and changes in attitudes towards care and support, moved care from long-stay hospital to individual homes and community settings. People said it would never work. Although independent self-advocacy groups continue to campaign for better treatment and person-centred services, the changes have happened. People do now live more independently than was possible in many of the long-stay institutions.

There have also been shifts in attitudes about anticipated quality of life for people diagnosed with cancer, people who have had strokes, people experiencing mental ill-health and people with physical disabilities. The changes happen when people become more aware, more engaged and less fearful. The stigma (shame and disgrace) attached to so many illnesses and conditions is removed through education and person-centred approaches that focus on putting the individual first.

Sometimes the stigma people experience becomes part of the individual's own thinking about their condition. Self-stigma erodes self-confidence and social connections, which adds to the stress of the situation. People who have recently been diagnosed with dementia may fear going out in case they forget what they went for or forget where they live. People may be concerned that they will become confused or behave in embarrassing ways.

There are many informative and supportive self-advocacy groups and networks dealing with these issues. The creation of dementia friendly societies and developing buddy, friendship or advocacy systems help address these fears. The self-advocacy groups are testimony to the strengths and capacity of people with dementia to show people what is possible.

If we meet a person in the later stages of dementia, a model I find useful to explore with staff and relatives is the Johari window, created in the 1950s by psychologists Joseph Luft and Harrington Ingham (Luft 1969). The model explores what we know and do not know about ourselves. I use it to show that we can never know everything about a person, which means we do not have the full knowledge to make assumptions. As shown in Table 3, there are four segments: Open, Blind, Hidden and Unknown (Luft 1969).

Table 3 The Johari window model (Luft 1969)

Open area	Blind area
Known to self and to others	Unknown to self, but known to others
Hidden area	Unknown area
Known to self but not to others	Unknown to self or others

- *Open:* This segment represents aspects of ourselves that we and others know about us. Our personal 'open' areas vary depending on what we share with friends, carers, colleagues and other people. Things we do and say (in public) are in this area.

- *Blind:* We may not realise how other people see our behaviour or personality. Sometimes our words or actions are misunderstood and we remain unaware until someone tells us. Equally we may not know how much other people value us. This area is about what other people know about us that we do not know. These become open when we know.

- *Hidden:* This is the area that we know about ourselves but other people do not know these factors. Our personal values, feelings, attitudes, hopes and fears reside here along with our secrets, undisclosed memories, motivations, unspoken regrets and desires. These emotional aspects move into the open area when we share parts of our hidden selves. It is from this area that we may behave in ways that other people do not always understand.

- *Unknown:* The last segment represents the things about ourselves that are unknown to ourselves and unknown to others. This could include the extent to which we can learn and develop, or the position we will be in a year from now, or the exact way in which a long-held ambition can be fulfilled.

Person-centred care can help move the desires, hopes and dreams of someone with dementia from the hidden area to the open area. This helps ensure individual needs can be met. The model windows shown in Table 3 are variable. For example, the more trusting or open we are, the larger the first window is. Likewise, if we become more aware of how others perceive us, this reduces the blind area and expands the open window. The bigger the open window, the easier it is for carers and staff to meet the person's needs.

People who are not easily understood by relatives and carers may have larger hidden and unknown areas. The issue here is that people often focus only on the 'open' window, which may not be very big, and they respond on that basis. The Johari model reminds us to consider all that we do not know.

Supportive and creative environments

No one knew very much about Nora, and she does not speak. The open window of the model was really quite small. However, when Nora's puppet taps its felt hand on the wall, the chair and the floor, people notice. Nora has been tapping her hand on her thigh and on the arm of her chair every week. It is almost hidden. Sometimes people notice the movement, but they seek to stop the tapping, perhaps thinking it is a sign of agitation. They hold Nora's hand until she stops moving it. They have not realised that the tapping is a way to connect with Nora. The moment they leave, the tapping starts again.

When a person's speech has gone, his or her body can still communicate. Nora taps away. One day a puppet that looks like her taps back. Tuned in to the moment, the carers notice this tiny exchange. The taps become a turn-taking activity – a call and response interaction. Nora stops tapping. The puppet stops. Nora taps three deliberate taps. The puppet follows. Nora smiles. The communication is subtle, but it expands the area where exchanges can take place and where relationships can be built.

Creating supportive environments can be as subtle as that tapping to large-scale enterprises. In the Netherlands, Hogewey Village is a care setting that incorporates the familiarity of a shop, hairdressers, café, gardens, separate houses and several clubs for learning skills or doing hobbies (Henley 2012). The purpose is to increase quality of life, and engage people in daily living skills, to maintain a sense of identity and enjoyment of life. The environment assumes people have the capacity to live fulfilling lives, and does everything to support this.

There are more such places springing up containing cinemas and theatres, libraries and pet corners. The future of care is creative and exciting! Carers are every bit as human as the people they care for. It is important that carers also experience moments of wonderment, connection and joy. Even a humble room in a domestic dwelling with one carer can still offer humour, validation, belonging, valuing, creative encounters, communication and love.

Over the years, it seems that although life purpose and roles are important, the closer that people live in 'wonderment', the less that seems to matter. Perhaps in the end, the identity we try so hard to maintain can be freed. Creativity, through music, arts and puppetry offers a bridge between the known and unknown, which helps us all connect.

CHAPTER 11

'Floby-dooby-do'

Stimulating Memories

'Floby-dooby-do...Flobby...Flobing-dobington...Fobby-flab-i-flab... Flipper Flob.'

The residents of a care home sit around a table talking complete gibberish and laughing loudly. It is a raucous introduction to the old puppets. Even people who rarely speak are joining in, and the noise level is high with laughter. The sight of well-known 1950s (British) puppets have generated such fun.

The television version of *Bill and Ben, the Flowerpot Men*, was created by Freda Lingstrom in 1952. The flowerpot men spoke a funny nonsense language and lived at the bottom of a garden (each inside a large flowerpot). They were identical looking marionette puppets, wearing straw hats. In the programme, their friend, Little Weed, pops up when they are not looking. The weed grows very tall, then she must shrink again before they return.

The 1950s and 1960s was a popular period for children's television puppetry. The majority of puppets I show are ones people remember watching, as parents with their own children. Many of the sessions stir memories of being a mother or father, as well as their own childhood experiences.

In another setting a lady calls out the name of a singing piglet puppet called 'Perky'. The marionette puppet walks towards her and she is thrilled. Pinky and Perky, the twin pig characters, were created by Jan and Vlasta Dalibor in 1957 (the rights are now with CBBC, the BBC's children's television). These cute pigs sang in high-pitched voices and had all sorts of amazing adventures! There were also popular Pinky and Perky annuals and colouring books. The duo released records (often cover versions). Many people recall Pinky and Perky's version of the song 'Would You Like to Swing on a Star?' (written by Jimmy Van Heusen and Johnny Burke in 1944).

In the care home, the lady delights in singing as many rude nursery rhymes to the piglet as she can possibly make up. She has the decency to cover Perky's ears before she swears. He is cradled on her blanket as she tells him exactly what little Jack Horner was doing in the corner, and why Miss Muffet ran away, and why the old cow was too fat to get over the moon. An unexpected reminiscence!

For years, care homes have engaged in reminiscence therapy, to help people remember their past, and stimulate brain activity. The story work in previous chapters helps capture, record and recall personal and cultural histories. The oral history society is an excellent online resource for people considering a history project. There are tips for interviewing and recording people. Libraries are also perfect places to do group reminiscence projects about particular subjects: transport through the ages; recipes; famous artists; fashion changes.

People enjoy discussing their experiences of major cultural events. During the past 60 years, changes include: rock and roll; reaching the top of Everest (Edmund Hillary and Tenzing Norgay); first man on the moon (Neil Armstrong); Berlin wall built and demolished; first human transplant (South Africa); Punk; Nelson Mandela released and the end of Apartheid (South Africa); Channel tunnel between Britain and France; the Olympics; and the Queen's Silver, Gold and Diamond Jubilee celebrations.

Group reminiscence can be fun, with quizzes or passing around objects of interest. The diversity and richness of life can lead to wonderful conversations. Friendships are built on common experiences. I met two men recently who were delighted to discover they had both lived in Korea. It often seems as though humans are searching for that which is like them. We recognise ourselves in other people.

Reminiscence work must be supportive to ensure people do not feel stupid or inadequate if they cannot recall the words. I once sat in on a quiz that had me gripping the arms of my chair in case I might be asked a question. The activities' coordinator had clearly spent a lot of time researching and creating the quiz. However, she was firing questions and telling people to hurry up with the answers. I asked my neighbour what happens if we get it wrong. He drew his hand across his throat!

Asking questions of people who are struggling to remember can induce more stress and exasperate the situation. It is important to maintain the light-heartedness of the event. The quiz coordinator relaxed when she felt more supported. Carers need to recognise when support is needed, and seek it or offer it, so the work can flow more easily.

Song words, poetry and the times table can be useful activities as seen in Chapters 8 and 13. There is also something about the rhythm or rhyme of rote learning that enables people to join in. Use activities that do not rely on forming new verbal responses, until the person seems relaxed and comfortable. Look at old magazines, hold vintage objects, play old board games as these can all stimulate memories.

Returning to the BICEPS model (Chapter 2), our priority is to set the Intention for having an enjoyable experience, using Creative thinking and Expecting some form of connection. The reminiscence may not be our primary goal, but the enjoyable interactions often lead people to recall more about their lives.

A group looks at the Sooty, Sweep and Soo puppets. Sooty is a British puppet (a hand puppet), with black ears and nose on brown teddy bear fur. Also made popular from the 1950s television, he began as a magician's assistant. Sooty held a wand and would whisper into the magician's ear (Harry Corbett), who said:

'Izzy Wizzy, Let's get busy!'

Sweep the dog joined the team, with his squeak and his long ears. This was followed in the 1960s by Soo (Sooty's girlfriend), who was a Panda.

The group members all recognise the puppets, and pass them around, inspecting them and laughing. A lady, who had been anxiously fiddling with her clothes, immediately reaches out for Sooty. The gentleman beside her helps to put the puppet on her hand, and they look at it together.

One man recalls pretending his child's teddy bear could talk to him like Sooty. The teddy bear would ask the child to finish his dinner, or go to sleep. People chat more and by the next session, family carers are asking what has happened to make their relatives start talking! People love the old puppets.

Andy Pandy (created by Freda Lingstrom and Maria Bird in 1950) is a marionette with a stripy blue and white playsuit and matching hat.

He lived with a teddy bear called Teddy in a gorgeous picnic basket. When they were not looking, a rag doll called Looby Loo appeared.

A participant recalled the song about Andy Pandy coming to play. She used to lay on the sofa when the children watched the show, so the song made her feel a sense of relief. Someone else asked why Looby Loo and Little Weed always had to hide from the male characters in the shows. This led to a discussion about the position of women in the 1960s. Many of the women in the group had gone out to work. Some had felt shame for not being 'good wives' who stayed at home.

These discussions and reminiscences help carers understand the lives and culture of participants. Staff or carers come up with more ideas for theme days, or activities. Discussions about occupations, equality, marriage, parenting and entertainment are initiated by an Andy Pandy puppet.

Muffin the Mule (playing the fool) was an earlier puppet. His head bobbed up and down (a lot!), but he was a much loved comical puppet on television. This was after the Second World War in the 1940s and 1950s with Annette Mills, who played the piano, and puppeteer Ann Hogarth. One lady said she hoped every Christmas and birthday for a Muffin the Mule toy. This led the group to create a 'most desired gifts' list.

Thunderbirds and Stingray introduced more sophisticated looking puppets in the 1960s. The puppet heads could change during filming, so they had more facial expressions. Stop-motion animation became more popular for programmes such as the *Clangers*. Another earlier version of this form of puppetry was the *Magic Roundabout*. People enjoy these comical characters, and can usually remember the character names.

One gentleman who rarely spoke became more vocal at home after the puppet sessions. He was delighted to meet Lambchop, an American ventriloquist sock puppet. She is a very cute lamb, originally performed by Shari Lewis in the 1950s (and continues with Shari's daughter). The Lambchop I have is still learning to be a ventriloquist puppet, but we were able to deliver a version of the song 'Anything You Can Do, I Can Do Better'. The gentleman nodded along.

A basket of sweets was passed around, and the man picked two. He unwrapped one sweet and presented it to the very white, sock puppet. Lambchop declined the offer, so the man popped the sweet in his mouth. He peered inside Lampchop's mouth, then took another sweet out the basket, which he unwrapped and presented to the puppet. Again she declined. He popped it into his mouth with a big grin!

More information about vintage puppets can be found in Blumenthal (2005).

Most television puppets like Basil Brush and Kermit have catch phrases or songs, which people often recall. Other paraphernalia can be found in second-hand shops. The puppets and books are a source of great fun. Some people had marionette puppets as children. The Pelham Puppets were particularly popular in the 1950s to the 1970s and sold in over 40 countries. More about them can be found on the Pelham Puppets website.[1]

Punch is *the* traditional puppet! He is perhaps one of the first puppets the majority of people I meet think of when the word puppet is mentioned. Mr Punch and his wife Judy formed a regular part of the entertainment culture for the English seaside, and are still going today. A single puppeteer performs the show, from inside a Victorian style booth (see Chapter 15). The words Mr Punch speaks are spoken through a mouth device (a swazzle) to create a comical voice. The audience can still decipher the words, although much of the event is slapstick.[2]

People recall the aggression that Mr Punch has for all the characters, as well as the comedy. The shows often depict one crisis after another, with strange twists and turns. Concentration lapses are not an issue, as within a couple of minutes, a new scenario is developing. This 'scene by scene' style of show can be very useful for working with people with short-term memory spans.

Hands-on, non-verbal reminiscence includes rummage boxes. Some museums offer a memory box loan service. Plan ahead, as there is often a waiting list. It can be better to create and decorate the boxes together. The box could be like the story box or memory box idea (Chapter 10) or as big as an old sea chest! Consider objects of meaning for the person if you know them well, or objects related to a particular theme or era.

In a care home, this also helps staff research the social history, and understand the cultural values of the time. A box representing the 1950s might have records, lipstick, knitting patterns, braces, model aeroplane kit, skipping rope, Wright's coal tar soap, ball of string, ball of wool, photographs, postcards, old coins and stamps. Items can be found on market stalls, or online markets and second-hand shops. Whenever possible use the real object or at least a photograph.

Notes

1. The Pelham Puppets website is at www.pelhampuppets.uk.com/pelham_history. html.

2. The history of Punch and other information can be found at the World through Wooden Eyes: www.theworldthroughwoodeneyes.co.uk/pob.html. Books on the Pelham Puppets, Punch and Muffin the Mule are on sale at the Mask and Puppet Centre, Glasgow: www.maskandpuppetbooks.co.uk.

CHAPTER 12

The Exotic Bird Comes Home

Animal Puppets

John rarely speaks with staff or visitors. Carers have not found anything or anyone that he connects with. People struggle to interact with him. He is younger than the other people living in the home, diagnosed with fronto-temporal lobe dementia. He spends time walking the hallways, and tries a few doors. He is agitated if anyone gets close to him, so the communication requires physical distance.

There is not much information about John; however, at the end of a session with someone else, I notice him watching the puppet dog. The dog 'runs away' and hides behind a chair. John initially appears to looks for it, then turns around and seems uninterested. But he suddenly spins around just when the dog puppet has re-emerged. The puppet dog (tied on a leash) jumps up and down, turning in circles on the spot. John smiles, then resumes walking alone.

At the next session, John is seated with a small table beside him. He watches the puppet dog, and seems to enjoy a repeat of the 'hide-and-seek' game. He turns his head to see where the dog might pop up next. There is no acknowledgement of the puppeteer or carers. His attention is only for the dog. That is until a big bright bird marionette puppet walks by.

John leans forward and watches intently. The bird walks past him again. John begins a gentle tapping movement with his fingers on his side table. The bird turns and moves towards the table as though looking for crumbs. John gently strokes the bird's beak. The bird starts to walk away, but the man taps his fingers again, attracting the bird. This sequence is repeated three or four times.

In between the encounters with the bird, John is moving his drink along his side table. At first it appears as though John is concerned that the bird is after his drink, so he moves it further away. However, as the scene unfolds it is evident he is making space on the table for the bird. He is planning the capture of this exotic creature.

Suddenly John reaches forward and takes hold of the bird's beak. He pulls the bird onto the table, carefully gathering up the body and legs. He tenderly arranges the bird. Not once does he seem bothered by the strings. In fact he slowly assembles the strings and the puppet control. Without looking at the puppeteer, he places these to the side, and arranges the bird's head to look more comfortable. When his task is complete, he leans back in his chair, then looks at the bird. His hand gently pats and strokes the sleeping creature.

This long and tender interaction happens without any words, and is very moving to witness. Animal puppets offer opportunities for people to show love and affection. It is highly likely John would have enjoyed real animals, but these were not present and he clearly connected with the animal puppets. We developed the work a bit more, so John became involved in puppeteering the dog. He usually wrapped the dog up and returned it rather than do anything else, but he loved watching it do various 'tricks'. (The dog could jump through a hoop, for instance.)

When I first used animal puppets, I was concerned they may be too childish for adults, but these puppets turned out to be highly popular. Many soft toys available today look remarkably real. Even those that don't (such as the exotic birds) still generate the 'Ahh' response. In many care settings people lack opportunities to offer the love they have.

Pet therapy is increasingly recognised as offering therapeutic or motivational support to individuals. I have witnessed increased social interaction and well-being when an animal is present. In a hospice a big soft white floppy rabbit would lie almost in a trance while being stroked. One care home had a large cat that purred extremely loudly when stroked. People with hearing impairment could feel the cat vibrating with those deep purrs!

Animals and humans have a long history of developing bonds, so it is not surprising that people enjoy having pets. Some family carers say the pet dog forms a special attachment to the person being cared for. Animals can help reduce stress and anxiety, unless they rip things up, soil the carpet, or hassle everyone for food all the time!

The pet therapy schemes offer animal visits with trained handlers who deal with potential issues. There may be an insured pet therapy scheme you can apply to. The animals can visit people in their own homes, in hospices and in care homes.

Some care homes have concerns about having real pets. This may be because of the extra work involved, but also because occasionally a person who is confused may be accidently rough with an animal. Some people may not be aware of their own strength, or trip over moving creatures. Animal puppets are the next best thing! The most popular animal puppets are the big birds (see the appendices) and cats and dogs, which are described below. The puppet animals can also be washed inside a bag or pillowcase in the washing machine at night, so there are no hygiene problems.

If you want your puppet to look fairly real, study how an animal moves. I look at head movements in particular. Notice the way a cat or dog moves its legs and tail. Making a kitten glove puppet may require a little surgery on fluffy toy kitten rear ends. Remove some of the stuffing, and if inclined, sew an inner lining. You want your hand to fit inside, with the index finger to the head, and the thumb and middle fingers into the front paws either side. If your kitten is more of a cat size, you can get more control with two fingers in the head, a thumb in one front leg, and the other two fingers in the other front leg. You move the back tail and back legs with your other hand.

Animating an animal puppet to pop up from a box, a bag or a hat is an ancient and effective way of grabbing attention. Our initial kittens had not had the surgery. Each kitten was animated by pressing on its back; this made the head move up and front paws splay out. I practised until the kitten's movements looked natural. The kitten lies beneath lots of bright pink netting inside a brown handbag with gold fastenings that clip and unclip with satisfying precision. Introducing a kitten this way seems to work really well everywhere we go. There is a shared 'discovery' that many participants adore.

Sitting with the handbag on my lap eases me into conversation with May, a lady in her nineties who had the sweetest face, and most graceful hands. She smiles and waves a hello to me as I approach. May is very quiet and self-contained, a lady with dignity. Staff tell me that May has an ornamental kitten that she seems to like. So with this snippet of information I prepare for my next visit with her.

Prior to this meeting, Helen, whom we met in the Introduction of this book, had already engaged wholeheartedly with the kitten puppets. Knowing the effectiveness of an intervention helps the carer or puppeteer know what is possible. While each person is an individual, there are certain puppets that go with certain people.

May asks if I have had a long journey to see her. I tell her the journey took me through a beautiful leafy lane, along a main road, over a bridge and along another lane beside a ploughed field.

'Oooh,' she smiles, 'What delights!'

I open the handbag and she immediately notices the bright pink netting. She reaches out and together we pull at the netting, unravelling the mass that has been tightly packed. She is laughing as yet more and more material appears. It is like an old magic trick with never-ending knotted silk scarves being pulled from the hat. May squeals with happiness at the sight of the kitten. She is keen to hold him. And there begins the most beautiful welcome any kitten will have received. No need to have rehearsed making it look real after all.

'Oh, there you are!' enthused May. 'How I have missed you. How I have wondered about you and searched for you. How glad I am that you have returned. Oh, my beauty.'

She holds him to her chest and strokes his soft body. I say I am wondering where he might have been. She looks at him and checks his bright, white paws. Much like Helen in the Introduction, May has a vast range of stories and imaginations. Perhaps she has memories of kittens.

'Well, I heard him scratching at my window in the night, and I was so worried about him. But he came to me, and I put a towel on the floor to clean his paws. I didn't think I could keep him, so I told him to shoo, but he would not leave me alone. And now just look at him! He is clinging to me!'

She holds him tightly, and we are both laughing at this obvious joy and warmth and excitement. It is clear the kitten now belongs to May.

On our next visit, kitten number two has had the surgery. She is inside the handbag beneath the pink netting and as we pull at the netting, I get my hand inside the puppet. This kitten likes having its belly rubbed, which makes it wave its paws in response. I ask May where her kitten is and notice she pats the lump beneath her cardigan. She reaches for my hand and places it on the soft toy kitten.

'Is he coming out today?' I ask.

May has a peek beneath her cardigan. She declares the kitten is not coming out at all because he has been up chasing mice all night. Later when I ask again, May lifts her kitten out briefly to rub noses with the handbag kitten. She gives me lots of information about how to care for the kittens, and says they need plenty of sleep. Sometimes her conversation enters other realms, but she returns to the kitten subject regularly.

On subsequent visits May's kitten is often asleep beneath her dress or cardigan. She explains what he has been up to. She speaks about the comfort and joy of having him back in her life. This lady, who does not appear to remember me, is able to continue the conversation week on week.

May's relatives are glad she made such a strong connection with something that brings her inspiration and delight. The kitten gives her an outlet for her love and affection. It is a means through which to communicate with her. One carer is concerned about the use of 'toys' in terms of them not being age appropriate. This can be an issue, and it is good to discuss such dilemmas, and ensure that the work is underpinned with respect.

If a carer regards the puppet as a children's toy, his or her own judgement and feelings of awkwardness will be conveyed to the participant. The pleasure then stops. However, if the carer is using person-centred principles, and unconditional positive regard, while also setting an intention for enjoyment, these issues disappear.

On our last session, May pats her bundle then points at my kitten. She sings a beautiful lullaby while stroking its head. The kitten falls asleep beneath the netting. May helps me shut the bag and waves me goodbye. She continues peering at her kitten and humming her beautiful song.

Conversation photographs

May took a great interest in seeing images of the kittens sitting on top of a bookcase, or among some flowers. She held the photographs close to her eyes, then talked about the time her kitten was found inside a boot! The animal puppets can be photographed in different locations to produce conversation starter images.

This could be an enjoyable intergenerational project where children and older people find familiar and unfamiliar venues for the animal puppets to be filmed in. The work inspires new narratives about familiar subjects. Sometimes we use photographs of real animals. People point out the type of dog or cat they might once have owned. This can be a sensitive area as people form very strong bonds with their pets. The animal puppet allows the same discussion, but they can also move the subject on if needed.

Animal drama

To enhance the surprise discovery element, make the animal puppet come out of various containers. This becomes more effective when there are materials to move out of the way, such as a basket with balls of wool and knitting for a kitten. Or a dog hidden in a basket with rags and items of clothing, The animal needs to have a personality, so decide if it is playful, naughty, funny, sweet or annoying.

A puppy puppet on a leash can be dragged around the room. Perhaps the puppy doesn't like walking, because he would rather be with the person in the comfortable chair. The animal dog might be made to hide and resist all dog whistles and name calling. But when the biscuit tin is rattled, or the person he likes calls him, he suddenly jumps in the air (when the carer or puppeteer pulls the string).

Puppies can be fixed onto skateboards or some other wheelbase for simple comedy effect. An even better comical outcome involves stiffening a dog leash with garden wire, so the puppy can now appear to walk ahead of you. It could pull you along in any old direction. Covering a bamboo cane with strips of material or ribbon and fixing to a makeshift harness has the same effect.

Dog biscuits could be hidden near people, and the dog must seek them out. These scenarios become mini-performances that some carers will be comfortable with doing and others prefer to watch. It may take some confidence to make a fool of yourself, and a level of awareness for checking how people are with the apparent mayhem. There is great pleasure in creating comedy with people who so want to laugh. Often we find people enter into the spirit of this mild form of clowning.

Carer feedback shows the positive interactions go beyond the sessions. People become more playful, more chatty or relaxed.

Further topics of conversation or ideas to enact can be found in animal books and magazines. You could experiment with drama or conversations about the following animal subjects: toileting, fleas, grooming, walks, paw prints, chewing furniture, scratching at doors and windows, barking, meowing, jumping, nine lives, breeding, pedigrees, chasing, catching things, being stuck up trees, getting under the floorboards, leather collars, leads and coats, names, vets, operations, teeth care, expenses, devotion, comfort and designs for a cattery or kennels.

Choose one or two topics, and bring them up as and when feels right. Sometimes the conversation does not go anywhere. But this is not a personal affront. Even if you did spend a long time giggling away as you prepared your scenarios and visualised the hilarious conversations you were going to have, not every topic appeals.

However, as we often find, the idea can work another time, or with another person. Just enjoy the connections you do make, and certainly have fun with animal puppets. Even a minute of fun and frivolity is 100 per cent better than none.

CHAPTER 13

A Sentence a Day

Incorporating Creativity into Daily Practice

Imagine care like this: Ann is a carer in a residential home. All the staff recognise that their work is about making connections for positive interactions and joyful experiences. The divide between care work and creative activities has disappeared. People know that using creativity in the work is beneficial for both the caregivers and the care-receivers.

Mornings are no longer just about helping people get up. They are about welcoming the day. Staff know how to centre and balance themselves through simple breathing techniques. This helps each person remember that his or her purpose is to create a positive atmosphere for people to wake into.

Bedside lights and soft music are switched on as a relaxing start. Calling cards and invitations are left on bedside cabinets along with a single flower, an interesting picture, an object, or a puppet positioned in a comical way. The day begins with something gentle, friendly and interesting. Staff might go out again, and visit someone else, to allow a few minutes for waking up. This is better than the shockingly rushed mornings of the past.

> *'But what about the time difference?' some care home staff say, 'Surely it takes longer to be all creative and lovely?'*

In my experience, allowing space for someone to find his or her way into the day takes about the same time as not doing that. Struggling with someone who is disturbed by the sense of pressure and urgency is time-consuming and draining. It impacts negatively on the rest of the day; everything feels harder. In fact many staff know this is true.

When staff develop a better way, they speak gladly of how they can ease the person into wakefulness.

If someone has been incontinent, there does not have to be a rush to whip off the wet pad or sheets. Allow a couple of minutes to form a relaxed and comfortable association. Speak about the weather or last night's television programmes. Establish friendly contact. There is no need to make the incontinence a big deal. Each task is approached sideways, so to speak, to allow the situation to unfold with ease.

Creativity can be part of daily caring, especially for people living with dementia, whose language and memory require more creative approaches. Creativity is not an additional task that only happens when the activities coordinator arrives. It is unfair and unjust for artists, puppeteers and activities coordinators to have all the fun! Carers are sometimes left to do the more serious work. Indeed, sometimes care staff have to deal with distressing behaviour that in fact the artist has inadvertently caused.

It behoves all visiting artists to understand and use the principles described in this book. They should identify and update their training needs to prepare the work to a high standard. For example, counselling skills training, dementia awareness courses, person-centred approaches to behaviour and risk-management training.

Ideally artists should also have some care work experience so they understand the environment and the pressures people face. Artists, including musicians and puppeteers, usually do make good connections with people, because this is the nature of creative process. However, they are with people for a relatively short time, and would no doubt struggle to sustain the joyfulness and connection for longer.

It is important that care staff gain more opportunities and confidence to use their own creativity and experience happier working environments. This is part of everybody's role in a care setting, and most carers we meet have amazing ideas to help change the culture and environment. We hear of carers bringing in ornaments or plants or music from home to brighten up the place. People can make care homes wonderful places to live and work in. There is much we can all do, even in the way we speak with someone.

In a domestic home, the carer does not have the luxury of different staff to share the workload, or help create the positive environment. They may be a one-man-band, who gets tired more quickly. It can be hard to feel motivated to do anything. However, creative approaches do energise people. Some home carers mention they have developed singing and dance skills. They have, what some describe as, 'crazy cat half-hours', where they feel uplifted by the freedom of creativity or music.

I have been describing creative interventions and puppetry ideas which can be used in any care environment. The events can be elaborate or simple, as described in Chapter 7 with theme days and celebrations. Some creative processes are very simple to incorporate immediately, and can improve quality of life very quickly.

Calling cards – a sentence a day

One of the calamities in care homes, or even in the domestic home, is that conversations tend to dwindle. When words become confused or the retrieval too frustrating, people with dementia may stop trying to speak. Carers tend to mirror this and reduce their conversational matter. This results in a steady decline in speech. Staff say they cannot think of things to say. Relatives say they find it hard to chat when there is no obvious response.

In some care homes the majority of sentences are directional or task orientated. The following seem to be among the most often used:

- I'll be with you in a minute.

- It's time to get up.

- Do you need the toilet?

- It's dinnertime.

- Time for your tablets.

- Move your arm/leg/foot this way.

- Open your mouth.

- Do you want tea or coffee?

Just *one new sentence* a day could make a vast difference to someone. This is a campaign I started a while ago, asking carers I meet to pledge a new phrase a day.

The calling card is to help people find that new sentence. In their pockets, each carer has a collection of ready-printed laminated cards. These have a subject (and possibly the carer's name). The subject is something the carer has an interest in. It could be a film, song, book, a topic such as pets, woodwork, clothes, computers, craft work, children's games, or what I saw on the way to work today, a meal I enjoy making, favourite plants, a joke – anything at all.

By leaving a calling card with a person in the morning, the carer commits to give the person a new sentence, as a gift. If the carer feels particularly chatty he or she may leave two or three calling cards with different people. This simple action requires nothing more than the initial making of the cards (they are collected after the sentence is delivered).

The cards are made from blank playing cards, and can be done with the care-receiver, or with other staff or relatives. If one new sentence a day feels too difficult, start with one a week.

The calling card reduces the stress of trying to find something to say out of thin air, or of doing the task to get a response. The person may respond, but they may not. The point is that the carer is offering something unique each day. This is as much for the carer's brain as for the care-receiver's.

One carer got into the habit of looking up short jokes from the Internet to bring to work each day. A man, who usually told staff to go away in the mornings, realised he was receiving a different beginning to his day. At worst he would groan about the joke, and at best have a really good laugh. This simple change of pattern made a positive difference to his and the carer's lives.

Another carer reported that after three weeks of saying a line from different songs, the person she cared for started mouthing some of the words at the same time. They were connecting. Of course singing can happen when undertaking any task, at any time.

The invitation

The invitation is another favourite creative idea. It requires some advanced thinking, but can become part of any occasion or event such as those described in Chapter 7 (e.g. an invitation to the museum, the art gallery or the book club).

On days when there is no planned elaborate celebratory occasion, something special can still be created. The invitation could be for any number of things happening that day. The person with dementia can be involved in the creation of an event, or helped to prepare himself or herself for it. Receiving an invitation creates something out of the ordinary. The event itself may be quite a regular thing, but changing the context promotes enjoyment.

Ideas include the following:

- An invitation to watch a television programme at (time) followed by a ten-minute discussion over supper. The 'discussion' might include comments on the character's personalities and dilemmas, the scenery, and what might happen next.

- An invitation to lunch in the café rouge at (time). Everybody must find something red (from shirts to paper to magazine images to bunting) to decorate the dining area. Part of the fun is in recognising things in a different context. People might like to wear something red to the 'café'.

- An invitation to visit Dr (name of local GP) in his or her surgery at (time and day) to bring the GP some cake and an update on your health. This offers a different slant to regular GP appointments, which can cause anxiety. The person can help tie a bow on the box or bag for the piece of cake.

- An invitation to dine by candlelight at (time). The preparations may include unwrapping fairy lights to be put up or folding napkins. (If hygiene is an issue, just use the folded ones as decoration and place fresh ones for people to use themselves.) Other preparations include writing menus, collecting meal orders from people for the cook, choosing the music for the evening, choosing formal dresses or suits to wear. There are some pretty battery-operated flameless candles and candelabras, if people have concerns over real candles.

- Invitation to try a new hair shampoo. Tie a ribbon on a travel size bottle of shampoo. Smell the shampoo, feel the texture of it, notice how much it lathers, and what the hair looks or feels like after. Give it marks out of ten. Decide how it could be advertised.

Invitations can be for anything. Everyday life events from folding laundry to gardening can be approached slightly differently. Being creative does not have to be all bells and whistles. Yet changing the context can make such a difference to someone's day. It offers opportunities for people to contribute, and to be the experts. These ideas link with Dorothy Mantle's concept of 'the mantle of the expert' (Heathcote and Bolton 1995).

> I consider that mantle of the expert work becomes deep social (and sometimes personal) play because (a) students know that they are contracting into fiction, (b) they understand the power they have within that fiction to direct, decide and function, (c) the 'spectator' in them must be awakened so that they perceive and enjoy the world of action and responsibility, even as they function in it, and (d) they grow in expertise through the amazing range of conventions that must be harnessed. (Healthcote and Bolton 1995, p.18)

In all the puppetry and creative events with people with dementia, we are entering imaginary worlds, and yet experiencing real joy, real self-esteem and real empowerment.

Quality time with each person

Sometimes carers say they have so many people to care for that they cannot give quality time to every person. This feeling can be overwhelming. Individuals generally want to give their best, but feel compromised by lack of time, lack of support, or lack of guidance. While with a person, the carer may be thinking of all that is not right with the job, or thinking about all the other people who need time and attention.

We do need better systems, better support and conditions for everyone involved in care work, formal or informal. Meanwhile there are things we can do within our means, right here and now. Here are some points to consider.

Know that you can spend quality time with one person at a time when you are helping the person to eat or dress or shave, even for a few minutes. Even if 19 other people are waiting, you can give quality time to each person when you are with them. Before you spend time with a person, remember to take a few deep breaths to focus. Offer the very best of yourself for the minutes you are with them. Know that you are giving the best quality care you can gather at that time. Offer your best eye contact, best voice, best intentions, love and kindness.

In those few minutes breathe with the person. Dedicate a sentence, a tune, a dance, a movement, a joke, or a silent blessing – something that is of the highest quality that you can reach in that moment. I have seen many relationships build on the sharing of quality minutes. It does not have to be done in great long hours of contact. We might pass someone in a street who smiles at us, and we feel good. It does not take hours to create that feeling. Many of the interactions and progress described in this book have been built on 10 to 30 minute periods *a week*.

In many care homes I have noticed a marked difference in the standards of care when staff take those moments to centre themselves before undertaking any task. Use the BICEPS principles to underpin your interactions and work:

- Breathe into the moment – be as centred and calm and comfortable as you can be.

- Intend comfort and joy – intend to create or share a wonderful time.

- Creative thinking – use imagination and inspiration to make connections or share creative activities as part of regular tasks.

- Expect a connection (beyond personal constraints) – go beyond the need to be remembered or liked and find the connection in the places of wonderment.

- Person-centred counselling principles – find the truth of the situations and feelings so you can be congruent, offer unconditional positive regard and respect individual needs. Have empathy and compassion.

- Self-awareness – recognise when you need support; acknowledge when you are making assumptions about a person; reflect on what seems to help the person you care for feel happy or comfortable.

Practise feeling good about yourself. The more you like yourself and appreciate your life, the more that 'feel good' factor reaches other people. Feel as good as you can about yourself. This means not beating yourself for not being able to offer 100 per cent quality care 100 per cent of the time to every person who depends on you, every day. Pledge a new sentence, or a few minutes of 'beingness' with the person. It is these small things that grow the difference. Even one minute of silent togetherness, even one genuine smile, or one gentle touch can make a positive difference.

Cognitive stimulation

Some carers may be in a position to support a few minutes of daily mental stimulation or learning therapy, as Kawashima (2012) calls it. (This was mentioned in the Introduction.) Kawashima (2012) suggests that reading aloud and mental arithmetic are two very effective activities for stimulating the working brain (the prefrontal cortex). This improves blood flow to the brain and improves memory. At the Alzheimer's Disease International Conference in London in 2012 Kawashima showed video footage of people becoming more alert, mobile, confident and creative within a month of daily brain exercises, with even more improvements a few months later.

Some of the positive change could be due to carers' increased meaningful contact, valuing and caring of people in a way that was not done before. However, magnetic resonance imaging (MRI) scans show larger areas of the brain are working after reading aloud and working on simple mathematics for 15 minutes a day 3 to 6 times a week.

There are so many wonderful ways to engage with these activities. The mathematics can be done verbally while helping someone to walk, or as a group exercise. Guess the number by answering yes/no questions, such as is it greater than five? Does it divide by two? Is it less than 30?

Choose a number (e.g. 12, and find as many different ways as possible to make 12 the answer to the sum, such as 4 x 3; 20 - 8; 2 x 6; 5 + 7; 60 ÷ 5; 5 + 3 + 4, and so on.

Where possible, make the activities have life meaning. Money can be counted for going shopping; or cutlery pieces for laying the table; counting calories; measuring out ingredients on scales. Ask people to help work out more complex, real life dilemmas such as the cost benefits of buying or leasing a car; or measuring a room to design a change of room layout.

For entertaining mathematics in later stages of dementia, sock puppets can do the times tables, opening their mouths wider on the answer to each sum. Start with the kind of times tables most people feel comfortable with: 1 x 2 is 2; 2 x 2 is 4; 3 x 2 is 6, and so on, or the 5 and 10 times tables. Build up to the other sums. People may not have had many opportunities to practise, so allow time.

Our Maggie and Rocky puppets also do simple mental arithmetic as part of their repertoire. They do additions and subtractions, or simply count items in a room. People with apparently quite severe cognitive decline often seem to enjoy these sums, and can do mental arithmetic more quickly than many care staff.

Create book clubs or writers' clubs and encourage people to read aloud. Many people with dementia read well, but are not given opportunities to do so. Additionally people's eyesight may have deteriorated but the issue may not have been realised. Try a magnifier to see if this helps and arrange to see an optician.

It is a lovely atmosphere when people take turns to read aloud for one another. People with dementia can read to carers or to local school children. Remember we are talking about 15 minutes in a day of mental stimulation for making a difference in cognitive function and well-being. Try poetry, favourite childhood books, magazine articles, newspapers, fiction and non-fiction. Find out what individuals find inspiring.

The books and mental arithmetic offer further topics of conversation. Part of the problem in care homes or isolated family homes is that not much happens for people to participate in. There are at least more technological applications for phones and computers to help stimulate people, such as 'old time radio' programmes; memory games; images and sound clips from the past. Television and radio can also be great sources of comfort and stimulation. People also benefit from social interaction and sharing physical activity.

Easy places to live in

Some care homes are using more of the ideas raised by Sir Gerry Robinson in 2009 about making care homes inspiring places to live. Ideas include everyday task-orientated activities. Have a washing line at a height people can reach, with pegs, a washing basket, and some washed clothes or bed linen. Have a car that people can wash and wax and polish. Prepare vegetables together at the dining room table. Fold the linen together.

Think of ways to help people access their own favourite things. One lady enjoyed music. She had a collection of CDs but could not open the CD covers. If her favourite CDs are placed on a velvet-covered board, with little rods for the centre of the CDs to go over, they are easy to see and pick up. If she has an easy to operate CD player with a photo showing which way to place the CD 'label on top', she can determine when and what music to play. An iPod may be even easier.

Help an individual see clearly what to do. Have door handles that contrast to the door colour so they are easy to spot. Place outfits that generally go together onto coat hangers to help a person know what to wear. Mark books with colourful stickers so it is easy for anyone to read a favourite passage. Have well-lit areas and interesting wall dressings.

Ensure a person has the best chance possible of finding the way to his or her room. Many a time I have visited a care home and not known which way to go because there were no clues or signifiers. In Stirling, the Dementia Services Development Centre (2012) offers excellent examples and advice for designing homes that people with dementia can live in more easily.

Not every person with dementia will need all these adjustments or clues. However, by making environments user friendly and dementia friendly, the world becomes more inclusive, patient, creative and supportive! Care homes and individuals in the community have the potential to be practical resources for one another. Creativity is a good way to build bridges and strengthen relationships through shared projects such as reading aloud, concerts, garden parties, and everyday arts.

Access to dementia friendly cafés, community groups, clubs or local services helps people feel more confident about going out. It is widely known that being more physically active helps increase feelings of well-being (Fox 1999). Staff in banks, shops and bus stations who understand the importance of patience, friendliness and giving clues, are making a huge positive impact on the lives of people dealing with long-term conditions affecting the brain; and their carers.

It behoves us all to live as healthily as we can. Longitudinal studies by Whalley (2012) suggest that people with dementia may have experienced a combination of physical, psychological and emotional critical periods in childhood and later negative exposures in adult life. If this is combined with a lack of learning opportunities and loss of coping abilities, enjoyment and resilience, the negative impact is greater.

Whalley's (2012) work highlights the importance of healthy living throughout life from intrauterine growth through to old age.

Healthy factors include dietary care, nurturing, nourishing, developing positive coping mechanisms, maintaining brain activity through learning and education, exercise, fresh air and enjoyment of life. These things seem to have a positive outcome on health and cognitive function, and can be enhanced in any care and community setting. While dementia research and assessments continue around the world, we must do the best we can to live as well as we can. One new sentence a day is a good start.

CHAPTER 14

It's Show Time!

Puppetry as Entertainment

'In there,' says a staff member, pointing to the living room, where 20 people sit in various degrees of slumber. Their wheelchairs and armchairs are arranged in a semicircle close to the walls. A television blares in the background. There are no staff in the room.

The puppeteers had explained to the care home that the show takes an hour to set up. But it seems the staff have been super-efficient in ensuring everyone is there on time. In fact some people have already been waiting for over half an hour. The puppeteers introduce themselves. They explain that the show will take a while to set up.

'They're here to fix the pipes,' says an old man who has spotted the bag of tools.

'Is it teatime?' asks a lady opposite. One of the puppeteers shows everyone a puppet to help explain their presence.

'How marvellous,' says a woman, clapping her hands loudly. This sets off a mild chain reaction of polite applause throughout the room.

The puppet is inspected in all manner of ways as it is passed from chair to chair. The residents respond with increasing enthusiasm and appreciation to every aspect of setting up the show. A frame is erected and someone claps. The cloth backdrops are fixed in place to more applause, so the puppeteers take a bow. A piece of scenery is positioned – there is a mild cheer. The level of laughter and banter increases to a party atmosphere. The stage lights are switched on to a chorus of 'Ooohs' and 'Ahhhs'.

As the clock strikes the hour for the show to begin, many people have worn themselves out. Others, who have been in the room for two hours, now need the bathroom. 'Oh, that was great fun,' says one of the men, vigorously shaking the puppeteers' hands as he leaves before the show starts.

The art of entertaining is a gift and a privilege. Audiences are generally kind-hearted and appreciate all sorts of entertainers. We've witnessed the love of jokes by plumbers and handymen too. This willing gratitude is a humbling experience. However, it is important to remember that just because people are in a care home or house-bound does not make them any less discerning. People know what they like.

This book has already explored the many benefits of using puppetry to work with people in care homes or at home in the community. Our final chapters look at puppetry in terms of entertainment. Chapter 14 is for carers, activities staff and puppeteers interested in delivering puppet shows. Chapter 15 describes how we enable people to create their own puppet performances.

Entertainment, in whatever form it takes, can be stimulating, enjoyable and relaxing. It can broaden our knowledge of the world and gives us a different experience from our daily routine. It can free us from our worries – at least for the time we are absorbed in the event. Boredom is one of the biggest problems for people being cared for, especially if they have never enjoyed solitude. For them the entertainment is a welcome relief. Some people gain pleasure from reading, listening to music, meditating, thinking or other personal pastimes, yet still appreciate the occasional social gathering that being part of an audience can bring.

Going to see a performance is a cultural activity. The experience can be enriching and enhances our sense of well-being. Good entertainment offers emotional and meaningful connection. It can also inspire further learning, keeping us involved in a cultured life.

Being the recipient of live entertainment offers a sense of being valued. People enjoy sharing the experience and laughter with others. It is possible to be part of the social scene in the audience, without the anxieties that other social gatherings can bring. There is less expectation to converse when being an audience member.

Puppet show styles are diverse and highly adaptable to different settings, for size and genre. They can easily cover musicals, comedy, drama and vaudeville variety acts. We have explored the wonders of singing puppets and the wide range of puppet forms. Rod and glove puppets are particularly flexible. I occasionally use a glove puppet character called Dr Doctor, and have great fondness for the simplicity of his structure.

Many people like the idea of using marionette (string) puppets. There is something fascinating about the complexities of manipulating a puppet through strings. It is a time-consuming, sometimes frustrating craft to learn, as there are more variables to consider. Strings do tangle and occasionally snap, but this does not have to be a disaster.

Our lovely Mr Dumbles puppet portrayed an overworked, past-retirement-age teacher. The string on his right shoulder had missed inspection and was frayed. Mr Dumbles was on stage in front of 70 people when the string snapped. His right arm and shoulder slumped awkwardly while he continued his performance. After the show, members of the audience said they thought the incident had been cleverly manipulated. Mr Dumbles' collapsed shoulder and dangling arm perfectly conveyed the impact of stress on teachers!

It is helpful to know that performance mistakes can be successfully accommodated and audiences enjoy having a unique experience. Adlibbing or improvisation is a skill to be encouraged to respond to sudden changes. For example, a puppeteer friend of ours had an accident with his Cinderella puppet in a care home. The puppet fell out of the carriage from a great height. The show took a turn and became a story about saving Cinderella's life, much to everyone's delight.

Fairy tales can be inspirational sources of amusement. Adults often enjoy revisiting childhood stories. The patterns of these old stories seem hard-wired in our brains, as mentioned in Chapter 7. We carry them into our adulthood. Each of us can find our place within a story and identify with the characters. How many of us have felt lost in the woods like Hansel and Gretel, or hoped to grow a magic beanstalk like Jack? How many of us have faced impossible tasks like those set by Baba Yaga?

Stories are relaxing; they can soothe and guide us. Story characters can have the most awful times, being locked in towers, or cast under spells, but they can recover, finding love and peace. They may feel as rejected as the ugly duckling, but later they discover the joy of belonging. Tales like this give us a sense of possibility and hope.

Storytellers and therapists such as Clarissa Pinkola Estes (1992) and Pat Williams (1998) have different approaches, but both promote the benefits of storytelling. Estes (1992) analyses stories, exploring which parts relate to our understanding of the world and ourselves. Williams (1998) prefers the stories to be told and left to do their own magic, kept whole and sacred. They share their knowledge of the powerful and healing nature of stories.

The fairy tales can also be adapted to offer another layer of meaning or humour. Perhaps Red Riding Hood realises something is wrong because her gran would never wear such a hideous nightcap in bed. In fact her gran is the least stereotypical granny in the world. Red Riding Hood decides to test the wolf, and he cannot possibly achieve what her gran can! So the wolf is discovered to be a failed imposter; he creeps off (planning his revenge on the three little pigs).

We have used traditional fairy tale stories and cabaret-style puppets, as well as more contemporary comedy sketches. Chapter 15 looks in more detail at storyboarding and script-writing to adapt familiar stories. Sometimes a performance needs to be shorter than a regular play, so people have the opportunity to see it from beginning to end. However, as noted earlier, it is our experience that people's ability to concentrate increases with practice and enjoyment.

We have found it useful to have a selection of five-minute scripts, which we can grow with the audience. The performance time can increase or reduce in relation to variables such as ill-health or concentration levels. Developing a series of self-contained sketches is ideal for offering the necessary flexibility. Carers who know the audience members can usually gauge the best time of day to deliver the performance(s).

Sets

Some shows do not require a set (puppet stage). It depends on the preferences of the puppeteer, the needs of an audience and the amount of time available for setting up a show. Our experiences have shown that even without any props, cloths or scenery, the puppeteers usually become invisible when a puppet is performing. This is partly because puppets are inherently magical, but also because the puppeteer's energy is channelled into the puppet. All life and focus is imbued into the wood or cloth. If the puppeteer believes the puppet is alive, so does the audience.

As a performer it is important to remain aware of what the puppet is doing at all times. If he or she starts moving too quickly or chaotically, it can actually make an audience feel motion sickness! The odd chase scene or comic effect anarchy is tolerable, but too much movement can make it hard for people to focus. Give the puppet time to be seen and appreciated. 'Less is more' when it comes to puppetry. Subtle movements, such as a slow turn of the head, make the puppet far more believable.

The script does not need to be wordy, especially if individuals struggle to decipher verbal language. People appreciate the opportunity to enjoy something visually stimulating. Scripts can be written to focus more on the body language and actions of a puppet. For example, the Russian puppeteer Sergey Obraztsov's show 'An Unusual Concert' in 1946 had stunning non-verbal characters (Obraztsov 2001). The show was a satirical exploration of poor performers. Audiences still find the film of the show highly entertaining today (available from sales@puppetstuff.com).

Where words are used, it can be useful to have scripts based on familiar language, such as the fairy tales or old song lyrics. Rhythm and rhyme seem easier for people to hook into. The old memory patterns recognise well-used phrases and this enhances people's enjoyment of the show. We sometimes ad-lib the scripts depending on audience response, so there can be more or less repetition and opportunity to participate in the show.

People diagnosed with early, middle and late stages of dementia seem perfectly able to focus on a puppet amidst other distractions. However, some people like to see a puppet set or an old seaside-style booth. This can help build excitement and be another source of joy. Brightly coloured cloth and decorations add value to scripted performances.

Some performers use pieces of cloth draped over poles. The poles might be held in a free hand, or clipped onto the backs of chairs. Puppeteer Andy Jones (2013) created scenery cushions used in his puppet shows in hospitals. Each cushion depicted a natural setting (e.g. a woodland, the sea or a hill) for the puppets to perform on. The hospital patients held the cushions, so the action took take place in and around the audience. Figures 5, 6, 7 and 8 illustrate some performance options.

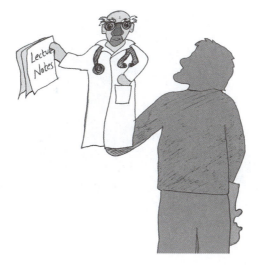

Figure 5 Free puppet, no set

In Figure 5, all focus is on the puppet. The puppeteer's energy is transferred to the puppet, so the audience becomes engaged with the animated character.

Second puppets are held behind the puppeteer's back when not in play. The puppeteer is free to move around. The use of props and where to put them can be problematic, but generally there will be a table, or a keen assistant among the staff and audience.

The cushions shown in Figure 6 could be adapted from regular cushion covers, or specially made for the set. By holding the cushions, the audience becomes the puppet set, and the performance moves around the room.

Easily recognisable as a puppet booth from the old Punch and Judy shows, the set shown in Figure 7 is usually used for glove puppets. The puppeteer stands inside the tent. The puppets perform on the shelf or playboard. Using a fancy frame for the window gives the booth a wonderful ornate look. This booth can be made by adapting a camping toilet tent. For a tailor-made fit, it is better to make the booth yourself. See the instructions at the end of this chapter.

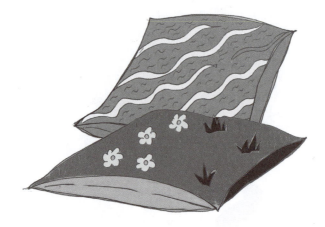

Figure 6 Cushion scenery sets

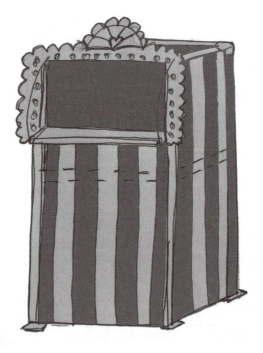

Figure 7 Seaside-style puppet booth

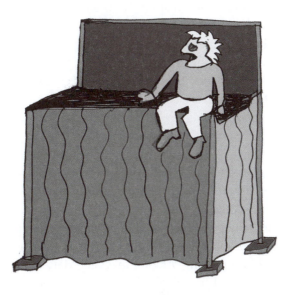

Figure 8 Simple booth for glove, rod, tabletop or mouth puppets

Figure 8 illustrates a simple booth measuring approximately 6½ feet (2m) tall at the back, 5 feet (1.5m) wide, with a front height of just over 4 feet (1.3m). The size can be adjusted as required. The front shelf (playboard) fits over the side bars. The puppeteer usually stands at the back and can see through the scrim material to the puppets, which are at face height. Rod puppets can be played over the top bar if desired. See the making instructions at the end of this chapter.

Our Dr Doctor short sketches have been done both with and without a set. The character works both ways. The glove puppet is easy to make (see appendices) with a papier-mâché head, big eyes, and bright colourful nose. Greens, blues and purples may all look alike to some people so, as explained earlier in the book, contrasting colours help people to see major features more clearly. Dark eyes on a pale face work well. Pastel colours are difficult to discern. We find that many people are attracted to yellows and reds.

Dr Doctor wears a white coat and always has a red stethoscope dangling around his neck. The sketches usually follow the format of him giving a lecture to a group of medical students (the people or person in the care setting). He has some non-verbal mini-sketches where we see him silently practising his GP skills, or having some sort of over-reaction to a little situation. He is a fairly pompous character, but people love him for his obvious blunders.

When being a speaking puppet, he usually appears charming and empathic, but can be highly insensitive. The scripts aim to be respectful of the audience members. Dr Doctor responds well to participation or heckling. He takes every comment as a point well made: 'a genius solution'; 'an amazing insight'; 'an intelligent comment'.

The puppet's name is immediately familiar because of the numerous Dr Doctor jokes. It seems that the love of these question and answer jokes goes back centuries. Mary Beard, a professor of classics at Cambridge, discovered that the Romans told such jokes over 1600 years ago (Flood 2009).

Apart from telling the odd joke, our Dr Doctor puppet (Figure 9) enjoys giving talks about his work. He delights audiences with some of the patients he brings along. Among them are Mary Mary (Figure 11) with her anxieties and Jack the Lad (Figure 10) about his new-found happiness.

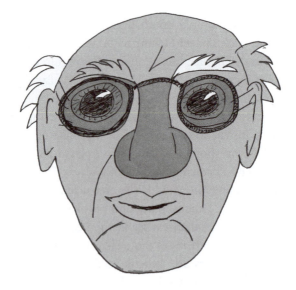

Figure 9 Dr Doctor

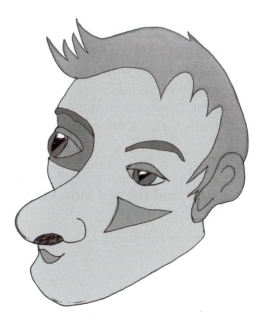

Figure 10 Jack the Lad

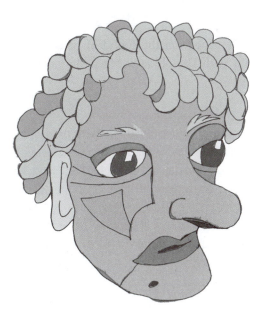

Figure 11 Old lady, Mary Mary

Copyright notice

Script 1: Dr Doctor and the old lady Mary Mary

Aim

Entertainment to enhance enjoyment using familiar rhyme with a different perspective.

Set up

For one puppeteer using two glove puppets. If performing without a set, the unused puppet is put behind the puppeteer's back. If using a set, the entrances and exits can be easier to manage.

Options

This sketch may benefit from the sound of bells and cockle shells to pass around at the end. The old lady Mary Mary could be played by a second puppeteer.

DR DOCTOR   *Enters in an upright, confident manner. Some small lecture papers are fixed to one hand. He turns to face the audience. Pats the stethoscope hanging around his neck. Clears his throat.* Good day to you all! I'm Dr Doctor. Thank you for attending my lecture. It is so good to see so many medical students here. Today's subject is about dealing with difficult patients. It is a sorry state of affairs, but we must learn to deal with them. I once met an old lady called Mary Mary.

MARY MARY   *Enters with head in hands (wearing a nice cardigan).*

DR DOCTOR   Mary Mary what a lovely cardigan. What seems to be the problem?

MARY MARY   *Crying (little jerks of head in hands)*. I don't have a problem.

DR DOCTOR   *Moves over to old lady and looks more closely. Moves away and turns back to the audience*. Upon examination I could see she was upset. *Turns to old lady*. Mary Mary, you seem upset.

MARY MARY   *Lifts head*. It's the bells ringing in my ears.

DR DOCTOR   *Moves back over to old lady and roughly looks in her ears. Moves away and turns to audience*. And I could she had little silver bells ringing in her ears. *Turns to old lady*. Mary Mary, you have silver bells in your ear.

MARY MARY   Well what will you give me for them Dr Doctor?

DR DOCTOR   *To audience*. I gave her some ear drops and sent her away.

MARY MARY   *Exits and returns with her hands on her heart and her head down*.

DR DOCTOR   *Does a double-take (is shocked that she is back so soon). To audience*. But she was back again. *To old lady*. Mary Mary, what seems to be the problem?

MARY MARY   *Turns away and keep head down*. I don't have a problem!

DR DOCTOR   *To audience*. How contrary our Mary Mary is. *Goes to old lady and prods her, looking at her from different angles. He moves away and turns to audience*. Upon examination I could see she wasn't right. *Turns to Mary*. You're not right Mary Mary.

MARY MARY   It's my heart…it's the muscles in my heart.

DR DOCTOR   *Returns to old lady and taps her heart. Moves away and turns to the audience*. But they weren't muscles – they were cockles. Her heart was full of cockle shells. *Turns to Mary.* You've got cockle shells in your heart.

MARY MARY   Well what will you give me for them Dr Doctor?

DR DOCTOR   So I prescribed her some ginger tea to warm the cockles of her heart and sent her away.

MARY MARY   *Exits and returns and falls down sobbing.*

DR DOCTOR   *Looks at old lady, looks at audience. Goes to old lady. Bends over to look at her. Moves away and looks at audience.* Well she returned in quite a state. I asked her, Mary Mary, what seems to be the problem?

MARY MARY   It's Georgie.

DR DOCTOR   Georgie? Your husband George? What ever is wrong with him?

MARY MARY   *Stands up and raises her arms.* He kissed the girls and made them cry!

DR DOCTOR   Which girls?

MARY MARY   Those pretty maidens who stand around all day in my garden.

DR DOCTOR   Oh. *He moves to and fro (thinking), then goes over to old lady and looks closely at her face. He moves away and turns to audience, lifts his hands; gives a big sigh. To audience.* She doesn't have a garden. *Turns to old lady.* Mary, Mary, you don't have a garden.

MARY MARY   Well Dr Doctor, why does everyone keep asking me how my garden grows?

DR DOCTOR   Mary Mary, I think the silver bells and cockle shells have caused a little mishearing and delirium.

MARY MARY   You mean?

DR DOCTOR   Yes Mary Mary. There's nothing to worry about. People just like to know how you sew such lovely cardigans. 'How does your cardigan go?' is what they're asking.

MARY MARY   *Opens arms and lifts head.* Well that's alright then. Thank you Dr Doctor. Exits.

DR DOCTOR   *Brings hands together then apart with a backwards tilt and 'hup!' as he returns to face audience again, hands apart then a quick horizontal karate chop (his sign to stop and listen).* Now dear medical students, I do hope you have learned how to deal with difficult patients. All you need is a little tenderness. My name is Dr Doctor and I have enjoyed the pleasure of your company today. *Bows and exits.*

The nursery rhyme in full:

> Mary Mary quite contrary
> How does your garden grow?
> With silver bells and cockle shells
> and pretty maids all in a row.

Script 2: Dr Doctor and the old lady's teeth

Aim

Entertainment to enhance enjoyment and promote discussion about caring for teeth. The participative nature of this sketch encourages movement exercise and laughter.

Set up

One puppeteer with one puppet. Props include garlic, toy false teeth, a toothbrush and tube of toothpaste; a mouth chart showing tongue, throat, molars, premolars, canine, and incisors; and a short pointer stick, such as those used by lecturers, fixed to the hand of the puppet (with an elastic band). An assistant or audience member is helpful to demonstrate what the puppet says, and to encourage further audience participation.

DR DOCTOR   *Enters in an upright, confident manner. He turns to face the audience. He pats the stethoscope hanging around his neck. He looks at the mouth/teeth chart, points at it with pointer, and clears his throat. He points to the audience.* Good day to you all! I'm Dr Doctor. Thank you for attending my lecture. I understand you are all training to be dentists and I am sure you will learn lots to help you along today. Let us begin with the mouth. This is the opening in the front of your face. Please check the location of your mouth, and notice how it opens and closes.

Assistant touches own mouth and opens and closes jaw.

Good, good. Now we will consider a few mouth problems that dentists have to deal with. Please open your mouths and say 'ahhh'. *Dramatically faints. Puppeteer prods the puppet who recovers and clears his throat. Looks at his chart and at the audience.*

As I was saying, mouth problems include halitosis, commonly known as bad breath, haggis mouth, dragon breath, sewer mouth, doo doo tongue and buffalo breath. Has anybody any suggestions for dealing with this problem? *Responds to any answers with affirmative comments such as 'genius', 'well said', 'good point.'* Yes, as dentists you can wear facemasks so you do not have to smell anybody.

The next problem you may experience is the tongue. Please locate your tongue and stick it out. Wiggle the tongue.

Assistant and Dr Doctor encourage tongue wiggling.

Good, good. Put them away. This second problem is very tricky. The tongue gets in the way of dentists seeing the teeth, so we must tie it up with a tongue twister. Repeat after me:

> Peter Piper picked a peck of pickled peppers.
> A peck of pickled peppers Peter Piper picked.

Repeat this as required with the assistant helping.

Good good. That will come in very useful as you perform dentistry. So let us move on to the names of the teeth. *Taps the mouth chart. Turns to audience.* Now, who can tell me the name of the big teeth at the back of the mouth?

Responds affirmatively to any suggestions.

Yes indeed. These are called molars. M – O – L – A – R. These teeth do a lot of grinding. The most posterior ones are called wisdom teeth. Dentists collect these teeth to increase their knowledge and power. If you come across anyone with wisdom teeth, whip the teeth out straight away. Do not hesitate, be decisive.

Turns to chart and taps it, faces audience. Let us consider the canine teeth. These are side teeth, and are also known as cuspids, dogteeth and fangs. You may know that fangs are one of the classic defining features of vampires. *Lifts the garlic and gives it to the assistant to show.* To keep yourself safe as a dentist you must pop some garlic in your pocket.

Returns to mouth chart and taps it, then faces audience. Before we demonstrate teeth cleaning, let us consider the subject of dentures. As dentists you will meet many people with dentures or false teeth. Each set of dentures has its own personality. For example, some dentures get tired and don't like to talk very much. Other dentures are complete chatterboxes. Some dentures like to go on holiday and will try and attach themselves to certain foods, or throw themselves out of the mouth with a sneeze. As dentists, you may need to offer counselling to some of the more wayward dentures. Does anybody here have stories about their dentures?

Responds in the affirmative.

Now we reach the teeth cleaning demonstration. First, we get our teeth in the right position. *Takes the pointer stick off the puppet hand and places the toy false teeth on the playboard/table.*

Next we take the lid off the tube of toothpaste. *Lid taken off by assistant or puppeteer and puppet.*

Then we get our toothbrush in position. *Place toothbrush near the toothpaste.*

Now we prepare ourselves to squirt the toothpaste. *Spends some time bending over the toothpaste, as though to squeeze it gently. Rearranges the position of the toothbrush. Moves away, then begins jumping up and down on the spot. Finally makes a run for the toothpaste tube and jumps on it to splat some out.*

Good good. *Takes a bow if appropriate.*

Now we clean the teeth like so. *Cleans the toy false teeth. For extra effect uses the wind-up toy teeth so they begin chattering around the playboard as the puppet chases after them with a brush.*

And there we have it! *Places toothbrush down and raises hands.*

Thank you for being such wonderful dental students. I am sure you will do well in your exams. Please give a big round of applause to *(assistant)*…for all the assistance today. I am Dr Doctor, and it has been a pleasure to see you all here. Goodbye. *Exits.*

Script 3: Dr Doctor and Jack the Lad

Aim

Entertainment that enhances awareness of some youth culture using common themes. This session could lead to further discussion about participants' own youth. Magazine images or old photos can make comparisons of fashion.

Set up

Two puppets for one or two puppeteers. No set required, although it might be beneficial to have a picture of a teddy boy to pass around the audience. There may be a lot of unfamiliar words in this script, as the youth culture language is being interpreted and translated by the Doctor. Some of the comedy is in the way the youth appears so awkward.

DR DOCTOR *Enters in an upright, confident manner. He turns to face the audience. He pats the stethoscope hanging around his neck, clears his throat.* Good day to you all! I'm Dr Doctor. I am happy as always to see so many keen medical students. Thank you for attending my lecture. Today we are talking about the well-being of young people.

I've brought along one of my patients. Jack the Lad! *Jack enters and stands awkwardly, head down.* Come along, Jack. Now you stand over there. *Indicates for Jack to stand about 30cm to the side of him. Turns to audience.*

Now when I was 17 we were wearing drainpipes with shocking pink socks. What a time that was! We had those drapes with the velvet collars – good for hiding bicycle chains! Oh yes! And I had a pair of blue suede brothel creepers for dancing – jiving and rocking to Little Richard and Jerry Lee Lewis. My hair was in a quiff at the front, with a duck's arse at the back. Held together with Brylcream! I had a slim Jim tie and a fancy waistcoat. Oh yes! The cosh boys we were called – we went around in gangs and the girls loved us.

But today we are here to learn about Jack.

Goes over to Jack and lifts his head. Stand up straight, lad.

Returns to his original place.

Good day, Jack.

JACK Yo Dude.

DR DOCTOR Hello. Now Jack, please tell us how life is for you.

JACK I is flatroofing 'n dry man.

DR DOCTOR So you are overworked and bored. Now Jack, tell us a bit more about how that feels.

JACK   *Looks around and shuffles a bit.* Me brain is clapping and I is vexed.

DR DOCTOR   *To audience.* His mind feels worn out and he's a little annoyed.

JACK   *Starts to sag and his head is down. The doctor goes over and makes him stand straight again, and returns to original place.*

DR DOCTOR   Tell me Jack, what does your mum say to help you?

JACK   She is so dread and grill bare nim nim nim nim init?

DR DOCTOR   She's not very helpful and talks a lot of rubbish – is that so? Well! Tell me Jack, is there anything good in your life?

JACK   I seen proper 'nang buff girl.

DR DOCTOR   Oh… *To audience.* He met a brilliant sexy girl.

JACK   Yeah dude, 'n she is lush bro.

DR DOCTOR   *To audience.* I do need to point out that I am not in fact related to Jack, despite him calling me his brother. It is just a phrase the young people like to use to establish communication. *Turns to Jack.* So she is very good looking?

JACK   'N jokes.

DR DOCTOR   And funny?

JACK   'N mint.

DR DOCTOR   And cool.

JACK   'N she got wicked shabby wear.

DR DOCTOR   Oh, so she likes to wear nice smart clothes! Well, well! And how do you feel when you are with this nice young lady?

JACK   I's buzzing now init?

DR DOCTOR	So you are enjoying life now?
JACK	Yeah bro, we is safe.
DR DOCTOR	So you are happy together, and all is well in your world. *Turns to audience.* Young love is so sweet, isn't it? All that innocence and lemonade.
JACK	And she is proper beast man.
DR DOCTOR	Jack! I really don't think we need to go any further. *Goes over to Jack and pushes him to exit.* Off you go now boy and behave yourself.
	Turns to audience.
	I do hope that has given you a little insight into the youth culture of today. In some respects nothing much has changed over the past 60 years. A bit less rock 'n' roll perhaps. They can't really do it in those trousers!
	I've enjoyed lecturing today. I'm Dr Doctor, and I expect to see you at my next lecture. Goodbye.

Building rapport

The scripts are short but strong enough to be repeated on different days. A rapport develops between the Dr Doctor character and the audience. Choose a main character you feel comfortable with, and create a back-story for him or her. This helps the puppeteer understand how the character would respond in any given situation. Scripts help the puppeteer maintain a framework from which to ad-lib and return to. This ensures a flexible response to meet individual needs.

Puppet booth making instructions

The size of your booth will depend on the following factors:

- The number of puppeteers to be accommodated.
- Whether puppeteers will stand or sit.
- Amount of playboard required for the puppets to perform on.

- Whether the puppets are played in front of the puppeteer's face or above his or her head (or both).

- How much weight you want the structure to bear (such as hanging props or scenery).

These directions show how to make a regular basic booth (see Figure 8) for a standing puppeteer performing with puppets directly in front of his or her face. A scrim curtain is used between the puppet and puppeteer to hide the puppeteer's face. The materials for the booth frame (Figure 12) can be found in hardware stores and through online supplies over the Internet.[1]

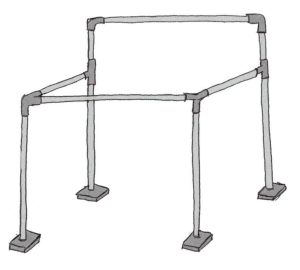

Figure 12 Booth frame

To build the frame you can use PVC pipes or rods. A diameter of 1½ inches (38.1mm) is robust enough for our work, but you could use 2 inch diameter for extra strength:

- 2 x 5 feet (1m 52cm) for across the front and back

- 2 x 4 feet 2 inches (1m 27cm) for the two front legs

- 2 x 6 feet 6 inches (1m 98cm) for the two back legs

- 2 x 18 inches (45.7cm) for the two side-width struts.

The feet of the frame are four pieces of plywood (6 inches square by ¾ inch thickness) with 1½ inch diameter holes drilled in the middle for the rods to slot into.

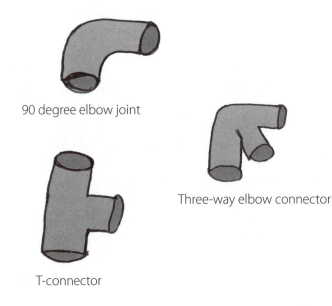

90 degree elbow joint

Three-way elbow connector

T-connector

Figure 13 Connectors

To connect all these pieces you will need the following PVC connectors (see Figure 13):

- 2 x 90 degree elbow joints for the top of the back bar to fix to the back legs

- 2 x three-way elbow connectors for the front legs to attach to the front bar and to the side struts

- 2 x T-connectors for the back legs to attach to the side struts.

For added strength you could add an extra front bar further down the front legs, so you would need an extra 1 x 6 feet PVC pipe, plus 2 more T-connectors (one each side).

If you wanted smaller diameter rods, go for fibreglass polyester rods: 10mm diameter is very strong and lightweight.

Curtains can be attached with Velcro over the bars. Scrim or dark gauze material is used at the back, so you can see what the puppets are doing. The playboard, where the puppets perform, is a piece of painted plywood which fits over the front frame. Strips of wood can be glued around the edge of the shelf, so it fits snugly over the bars. More strips of wood or ornate wood moulding can be glued to the top edges of the shelf. This provides a lip to prevent props from rolling off the mini-stage.

The seaside-style puppet booth (Figure 7) is along the same principles as above. If making a 3 foot square booth, you would need 4 x 7 feet lengths of PVC pipe for the height, with 4 x 3 feet pipes for the top of the frame, attached to the lengths with 4 x three-way elbow connectors.

Add more 3-feet struts on three sides of the tent about halfway down and again at the bottom, using T-connectors. The back wall is left so you can get in and out easily. The playboard is a piece of plywood with a lip that hangs over the bar. This is held up by a chain on each end of the shelf, which is attached to the bar at the top of the tent. The window surround can be a lightweight picture frame or made up of wood trim mouldings. Enjoy finding the right material for the tent. A roof is not needed, so you can breathe OK!

Note

1. Apart from local hardware stores, there are online resources, for example PVC pipes are available at www.cityirrigation.co.uk, PVC connectors can be found at www.formufit.com; other sources include Amazon and eBay.

CHAPTER 15

I Did It My Way

Puppeteers Who Live with Dementia

Janet is wearing a big purple hat and sparkly scarf, as she dances with her large marionette bird. The bird has bright ear-rings and a fluffy pink boa. The audience loves the dance routine and at the end Janet takes several bows.

Six weeks earlier, Janet was a tentative participant, but her humour, mobility and love of colour quickly became apparent. At the end of this creative learning programme, people have the option of performing with puppets, as actors, dancers or puppeteers. Although she was nervous, Janet chose to work on a choreographed dance and puppet routine. The simple animal and bird marionettes are perfect for this, as their innate humour help relax the performers and audience.

Larry, who is wearing a top hat and bow-tie, does his dance routine with two other men, each with comical dogs on sticks. Part way through the music Larry seems to lose the timing. He does what he can to follow the other men. They move in front of him, partly to show him what to do, and partly to hide his mistakes. Larry takes this as an attempt to steal his limelight. He abandons the puppet dog, walks in front and launches into an ad-lib dance with hip twists, which is extremely funny. At the end he shouts:

'I did it my way!'

Participative performance

Much of the work described throughout the book involves people living with more pronounced cognitive decline. They have experienced changes in communication or respond less noticeably to the environment. The creative process, including performance, can be adapted to suit people with a wide range of abilities.

Participative performance takes the pressure off the person with dementia. They do not need to lead or remember the whole performance, but must have opportunities to be included. The dance and puppet routines are good examples of this, where staff, artists and people with dementia share the performance.

People have stories to tell and ideas, plans, dreams, memories, thoughts and feelings to express. These do not have to be in words for the performance to be effective. Think of emotions and inspirations we perceive through works of art or music, without necessarily knowing what the artist or painter means.

Performance art also lends itself to conveying strong and direct messages to the general public, schools or peers. One of the main messages our programmes convey is that people are more than labels or diagnoses. There may be particular subjects people wish to communicate, such as reducing the fear of dementia; increasing positive attitudes; reducing stress in life; understanding how the brain works; understanding how it feels to care or be cared for at home, and so on. These can be done 'one step removed' through the puppets.

The genre of the performance may be dictated by individual personalities. I enjoy finding comedy aspects, although the poignancy of a piece is often present. Staff need to maintain awareness for whether the participation in performance is uplifting or likely to cause distress. Some people argue for a representation of 'real life' drama, including hardships, loss and sadness. My concern is that to focus on these areas can be counter-productive. But, if performers would like to tell their stories through performance for cathartic release, the process can be supported.

In my experience, people may begin with the traumas or sense of disempowerment; telling stories about difficulties, heartaches and illness (all of which can impact negatively on health). They may also speak about redundancies, financial hardships, divorce, fires, floods, daily life frustrations, fears, anxieties and dementia. However, the creative process seems to quickly allow people to recognise their strengths and qualities.

The work can be presented with humour or from the perspective of a celebration of individual strength and survival. It can also be presented with messages for potential resolution.

We have regularly seen that staff gain fresh insights and revise their approaches to people following creative expression. For example, one gentleman who no longer spoke used his puppet to convey his love of being outside and gardening. The puppet grew livelier when it stepped off the painting of a living room, onto the painting of the garden. Whether the performance is a minute or an hour, the impact can be profound.

The following participative puppetry piece is based on stories of loss and forgetfulness of people with dementia. It is comical, although here on the page it appears more serious than when it is performed. It can be done anywhere (at home, in a care setting, on a bed). Participants seem to connect with the puppet who is inconsolable at the beginning.

The staff/carer/puppeteer uses a hand puppet (see the appendices for making one). The puppet appears hunched up with his hands covering his face. When he rubs his eyes, and his 'shoulders' heave up and down, we recognise the body language of someone sobbing and know he is very sad. He has lost something.

The puppeteer taps the puppet on the shoulder and presents him with different articles. These are the sorts of things that people regularly misplace in their lives, such as keys, money, comb or mobile phone.

The puppet becomes increasingly distraught as each article turns out to be the wrong thing. Perhaps the puppet lays down and has a tantrum, or turns his back on the objects. With each tap of the shoulder he just about calms himself to look expectantly at the next object, only to find it a great disappointment. He silently wails and rushes into walls or grabs bits of clothing to blow his nose. These exaggerated movements are humorous, but also moving.

Often the audience member seeks to offer an item in their possession – a tissue, a hairgrip, a biscuit. At home there is usually more to offer than in a care setting, but one gentleman made a little hat out of a corner of the newspaper to give to the puppet.

At some point in the scene, either the puppet receives the thing he most wants (in this case the hat), or he abandons all gifts and instead clasps the hand of the audience member. He lies down in the hand of the audience member, to go to sleep. (This can cause the puppeteer wrist-twist so be creative with positions!)

The short performance seems to develop the participative elements on second and third showings with the same audience member(s). People volunteer to show the puppet more things. The ending is either the joy of finding a lost object, or the peace of a caring and loving hand.

Patterns or rhythms in participative arts are important as indications for people to latch on to. When building a performance over several sessions, it can be helpful for participative performers to work with the same partners to build familiarity. This is not always possible, so the pattern – such as steps to a dance or choreographed movements – becomes more important.

Life stories and messages can be developed into mini-musicals or cabaret acts that have the pattern of songs, catch phrases or short turns. The more quirky the performance, the easier it can be for people to get involved. When participants wear big hats or glamour clothes, their inner diva or film star appears.

There is a camaraderie that builds between performers, whoever they may be. The anticipation of the event and the thrill of the performance deepen connections between people. There's no business like show business!

Skills required for performance work

People are often more talented than they give themselves credit for. Individuals with dementia have a wide range of skills and abilities, experience and knowledge useful for performance work. Sometimes, there is an added advantage in terms of being less inhibited, or more willing to give things a go. Although extra time may be required for learning phrases or routines, the end results can be astounding.

People discover they have natural aptitude for comedy; singing; dancing; acting; puppeteering; mime; narration; or playing musical instruments. The beauty of creating a show is that it involves diverse talent:

- story-making and script-writing
- design of the set and puppets
- production and making of the puppets and scenery
- sound

- costume design and costume making

- props

- stage management

- lighting

- director and producer roles

- marketing and publicity

- front of house.

Classics, plays and musicals

People may prefer to produce a ready-made play. You could commission local playwrights to work with the care setting and create a relevant piece of theatre. Or you could use an off-the-shelf play such as Shakespeare (which does not need copyright fees). Royalty fees are payable on a scale, and as a care home or amateur dramatics society, the fees are less than for professional companies. A royalty is usually due when any part of a play is performed in front of any size audience, whether or not they are for profit and whether or not the audience buys tickets. These fees apply to music or songs too.

The advantage of doing a classic play or musical is the familiarity of it. People often already know parts of the script or the musical numbers. There are organisations that supply scripts and scores for plays and musicals. These include the royalty fee. There are also royalty collection bodies who pay the artist (see the end of this chapter for useful websites and addresses).

Local musicians or participants may donate their own music and songs to the show. (This is a gift we have been very fortunate to receive for some of the projects.)

Our process

In professional theatre, our work may undergo intense periods of production and reviewing. Sometimes in the past, the show has undergone whole remakes before the performance is ready to tour. This can feel chaotic and uncertain. Longer thinking and planning stages can help the process run more smoothly.

When working with people whose thinking, concentration and communication are affected, we do our best to maintain a higher level of consistency. This helps to reduce confusion and stress.

It is important the process is achievable and meaningful. A whole team approach helps the production and performance in care homes succeed. The first sessions are necessarily fluid, to find out what people are interested in creating. We use a story-making process based on themes raised by the participants.

For example, the narrative to puppetry work (shown in Chapter 7) used the theme of the sea. The area is close to the sea so people may have common experiences or personal history of the subject. Individuals are given paper marked into six squares and asked to draw stick images of the following:

- the main character in the story who lives near the sea

- the sea (rough, calm, stormy, dark, pale, frothy, deep, shallow)

- the mission or occupation of the main character

- something from the sea that stops the person achieving their mission or occupation

- something or someone that helps the person overcome the problem

- and how the story ends.

In more than ten years of using various story-making processes with hundreds of adults, I have not seen two stories exactly the same. This provides a rich source of story work to create performances from. Sometimes the group amalgamates different stories into a larger tale. Most often there is a story that several people feel resonates with them, and so they share in the production of it.

We establish that the participants, staff and facilitators are one production team. Photographic and video consent is requested and a photographer from the participants or staff team is appointed. There is an opportunity to experiment with and discuss ideas, images and desirable phrases. This helps people build confidence and gain more understanding of the different elements they would like to be involved in.

There is a lot of creative work ranging from searching through magazines for images to create a scrapbook of ideas for the show, to designing the sets, creating character lists and gaining a better sense of whether the puppets need to be shadow puppets or more physical puppets.

It is always useful to have a production manager with a clipboard and pen who can list ideas being generated during the first few sessions. Questions on a flipchart can also help people decide what sort of show they would like to aim for:

- What excites me about this show?

- What is the show about?

- What might this be about if it was a metaphor?

- Is the show one story or a series of acts?

- Does the show have any musical numbers in it?

- Does it have a happy ending?

- Which characters could be funny or happy?

- Which characters could be scary or unhappy?

- Who is the show for? Age range?

- Does this show have a message? If so what is it?

- Where and when will the show(s) take place?

- Do we need light and sound systems?

- How will we know if it is any good?

Some elements may require a voting system or a decisive director to clarify the final aims.

Our script-writing, puppet-making and set design happen in correlation to one another. The basic story layout and sketches can be transferred to a larger storyboard. The bigger the better, so people can see clearly what is required for the show. A storyboard (often presented like a cartoon strip) shows what the characters are doing and their physical location throughout the story. This informs the number of scene changes required and what the puppets or performers need to be able to do.

Some adaptation is often required to the script or for the puppets and performers to make the show work. Once the group knows what it needs, assistance can be requested from the local community to source props and materials. Community involvement and intergenerational work is also important for breaking down barriers and reducing stigma. People with dementia producing their own show helps the general public see beyond the diagnosis.

Sometimes care home staff have concerns about health and safety or adult support and protection issues. These can all be negotiated. Identified risks can be planned for and managed to minimise the likelihood of accident or harm.

Detailed planning of the production tasks enable carers, the people they support and community members, to work together for specific outcomes. It is important the work is shared rather than people doing things for people with dementia. For example, we check how every task can be made accessible. Puppet parts can be temporarily nailed to a thin board from beneath to hold them steady for painting. Desk easels can be made for easy sight and reach. Backdrops can be painted using thick paintbrushes tied to long sticks.

While some people enjoy designing the marketing materials (posters, flyers, press releases and so on), this could also be a project for a local school. Children can bring their ideas to the care home, and the people choose which posters they want to use.

Rehearsals need to be relaxed, creative and fun to help people feel at their best. If a particular scene is not working with the puppet or performer, explore whether it needs to be done in a different style, or how it can be better supported. If the puppeteer needs direction to make the puppet perform better, talk to the puppet. This helps establish the puppet as the main focus, and is less stressful for the person being directed.

Similarly, if a performer is playing a character, and needs instruction, talk to the character rather than the actor, so it isn't so personal. The photographer and film person can help by recording images and scenes, which can be printed and used as rehearsal reminders. If people feel anxious about recalling their words, audio recordings can be used as a back-up. The puppeteer or performer is still on stage but with a voice-over.

Build clues into every aspect of the performance. Sound and lighting can be used as prompts. Tape on the ground can help people know where to stand. Co-performers can work alongside each other or within eyesight of each other. We often find people create positive ways to support one another.

Rod puppets sometimes work better with two puppeteers – one to control the head and arm, the other to make the feet work. This pairing offers excellent opportunity for discreet support.

Before the main performance it is usual to have dress and technical rehearsals. These can be exciting as well as daunting moments for performers. Offer as much positive feedback as possible. Make final changes as required. Be prepared for all eventualities. We once performed a show in a city theatre with a group of people we had been working with for three months. The TV cameras were there, and one hour before the show one of the performers needed to pull out. We had made the show flexible enough to cope with significant changes. The audience did not realise there was an issue, and the show went well.

It is important to meet after the performance. The process of producing and performing a show brings out a variety of new perspectives. It is helpful to identify and acknowledge insights and learning, to see how these can be translated into better care practice.

It is natural to feel a sense of anticlimax following a performance. But this is just a dip in energy after such an adrenaline rush. The follow-up can highlight positive aspects and generate ideas for future projects. Having a visual record of the show is useful for this purpose, although not everyone will recall their part in the show, the feelings of being part of something special may remain.

Puppetry has an innate special quality that connects on an emotional level. Puppets are comical, but they also have a sense of dignity and respect. Sometimes we think we are making a particular character puppet, but it turns out to be quite different. An early puppet that was to play a meek and mild character gained a presence that startled the puppeteer each time he passed it sitting on a chair. Another puppet that was meant to be fierce and angry moved in the most endearing and hilarious way.

Puppets do not always do what is expected of them. A leg may fall off, a head might turn and face the wrong way, and the beautiful leading lady could fall off stage. This is part of the attraction of them. People who create puppets of their selves are creating something quite magical and inspiring.

Table 4 Do's and don'ts of using puppets in care settings

Unhelpful things	Good things
• Do not use puppets in a childlike fashion (e.g. speaking in baby language or being condescending) • It is not good to waggle puppets in someone's face • Do not rush up to anyone with a puppet • Never use the puppet to threaten anyone • Try not to jiggle a puppet around too much as it is hard to focus on • Do not use the puppet to ridicule a person • Do not have chocolate around puppets	• Allow time for a puppet to be seen • Less is more in terms of movement • Respect individual creativity and unique approaches to participative arts and puppet-making • Seek and acknowledge positive puppet characteristics or performance • Assist individuals to create what they want to • Allow time for people to be with their puppet without demands to perform or respond in any way • Ensure all making is made accessible and achievable • Use washable materials for animal, sock and glove puppets if sharing • Use antibacterial wipes on hands or inner gloves for hand puppets or controls • Treat the puppet with respect

Ensure the work offered to participants is at the right level. If the activity is mentally complicated or physically difficult, there is a risk of people feeling de-motivated, fearful or frustrated. Prepare the work to suit a variety of circumstances and abilities. For example, we create puppet parts in the following stages:

- uncut wood with desired measurements, a clamp, gloves and a saw

- ready-cut wooden shapes needing to be sandpapered

- heads requiring features

- finished wooden shapes needing to be painted

- finished/painted wooden shapes needing to be put together
- put-together wooden puppets needing to be dressed/decorated.

The materials, tools and instructions for each of these stages are presented clearly in ways to suit the individuals (verbally, pictorially, physical examples and in writing). It is important that all creative activities allow and support individual creativity. This means ensuring there is a choice of colour, material and sizes. In later stages of dementia we may be noticing which objects or colours a person looks at the most, or notice their own style of dress. We offer likely favourites with one or two other choices. If eyesight is an issue, we ensure the person experiences a choice of textures and describe the materials to them.

The making of a personal puppet is an important part of our narrative work. There is natural progression into script-writing and mini-performance work.

One of my favourite moments was watching two quite separate older ladies make cartoon puppets of their selves that interacted through the model theatre. There was a moment when they looked at each other and smiled the smile of deepest recognition and joyfulness. Their puppets were standing side-by-side, one dressed as a princess, the other as a policewoman, being who they said they wanted to be.

My hope is that the experiences and stories given in this book have resonance with you. All the people represented here have given something very special that increases awareness and understanding of living and dying well. They have shown us how to connect through puppetry and joy. The creative work is underpinned by an understanding of humanity that we can all share. Some of the concepts may require second readings to fully appreciate the meaning held here. Dementia care is about relationships, but not as we have known relationships to be. The connections seem to go beyond the personal, into the realm of creativity in a place that is *now*.

May you have many happy encounters on your travels beyond alienation into wonderment.

Useful information about royalty fees

Pioneer Drama Service

Pioneer Drama Service has a supply of over 900 plays and musicals with royalty fee prices shown at the time of purchase. They include the classics and also offer guidance and support. Based in Colorado, USA, the Pioneer Drama Service has distribution in the UK, South Africa, Australia and New Zealand.

www.pioneerdrama.com

Hanbury Plays

Hanbury Plays has over 300 plays, including classics. It gives royalty fee quotations when you complete a form that explains how many performances you would like to do, and the size or audience capacity of the venue.

www.HanburyPlays.co.uk

Performing Rights Society (PRS) and Phonographic Performance Ltd (PPL)

I have found both the PRS and PPL extremely helpful on the telephone to discuss what we are looking for and potential costs. Musicians and songwriters register their music with the PRS or the PPL. PPL represents record companies and performers. PRS for Music represents composers, songwriters and music publishers. These organisations collect fees for production music for creating DVDs, or for using music in a venue before and during the play.

www.prsformusic.com
www.ppluk.com

Cue sheets

It is important to keep a record of the sounds, musicians and songs being used for the performances. Some venues also hold licences for playing music publicly, and would need to have a copy of the list of music you intend playing (a cue sheet). The cue sheet contains the following information:

- Name and address of the project, company or care home

- Cue number, e.g. Number 1 song, Number 2 music, Number 3 song

- The title of the song, who the composer or songwriter is

- Which society the royalty fee is payable to

- What the music is being used for, e.g. background or visual live performance

- Timing (length of music being used, and what part).

We also use the following companies to buy original royalty free music. The music still belongs to the composer, but we purchase a licence for a one-off fee:

- Premium Beat: www.premiumbeat.com

- Royalty Free Music: www.royaltyfreemusic.com

- White Beetle: http://whitebeetle.com

Useful information about copyright myths can be found here: www.premiumbeat.com/blog/music-copyright-myths

How to Make Model Theatre Puppets

The model theatre puppets are made out of cardboard. This activity can be quick and easy to share. It is used with narrative or life story work. More in-depth making can be done by making the model theatre.

You will need

- drawings or magazine images of people approximately 15cm tall
- cardboard
- glue
- scissors
- sellotape
- strips of card or garden sticks approximately 15–20cm in length
- self-portrait images or photos approximately 4cm squared.

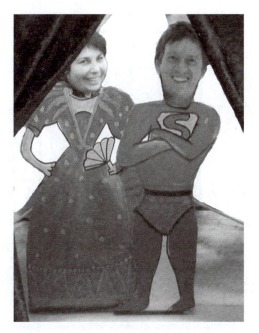

Figure 14 Cartoon figures

Directions

1. Draw or find images of people in various positions and places, wearing different clothes, doing diverse occupations or hobbies. A good size is approximately 15cm tall when standing (see Figure 14).

2. Glue the people images onto cardboard and cut out, leaving a lip on the base, which helps the character stand.

3. Draw or use copies of photographs of the individuals' heads. These can be approximately 4cm square and are usually big in proportion to the available bodies.

4. Choose appropriate bodies for taping or gluing the heads onto.

5. Sellotape the cardboard strips or sticks sideways onto the bodies, for whichever side the puppet will be controlled from.

These puppets become more effective when framed in a model theatre (see Figure 15) with backdrops and side panels. Storyboards can be made from the narrative, listing all the main characters and the scenery. The making can be as simple or elaborate as desired.

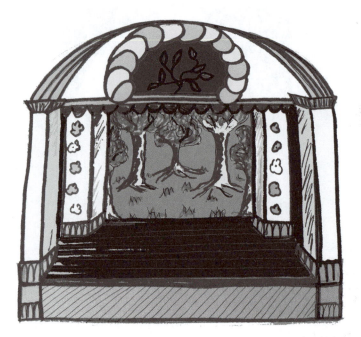

Figure 15 Sketch of a model theatre

How to Make Singing Sock Puppets

Odd socks can usually be found at the back of sock drawers! Use any colour socks to create these simple but effective puppets. To use the sock puppets for singing, see Chapter 8.

You will need

- one clean sock per person
- cardboard mouthpart shaped as shown in Figure 16
- two buttons or felt eyes and glue
- cardboard tube
- marker pen
- wool, netting or other fabric for hair
- material scraps, lace, ribbon and leather
- scissors
- needle and thread
- optional sleeves cut from old shirts or scarves to cover the arms if the socks are short.

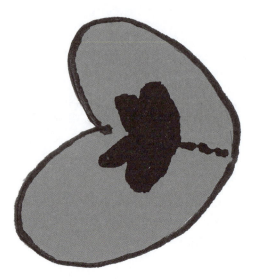

Figure 16 Cardboard mouth shape

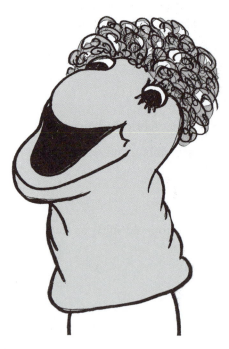

Figure 17 Sock puppet

Directions

1. Place a sock over your hand. Four fingers held together make the top of the mouth, while your thumb makes the bottom. Practise opening and closing the puppet's mouth.

2. Use the marker pen to mark the position of the eyes, hair and the back of the mouth.

3. Bend the cardboard to ensure it fits in the mouth. Mark its position.

4. Remove the sock from your hand and place over a cardboard tube for ease of access.

5. Cover the cardboard mouthpart in red material or a colour that contrasts to the sock.

6. Now carefully glue and sew this onto the mouth of the sock. (The cardboard fold matches where you marked the back of the mouth.)

7. Sew or glue hair, beards and moustaches in position, and add other features as desired, such as bow ties or hair ribbons, a scarf or hat (Figure 17).

How to Make an Adult Glove Puppet

The glove puppet is a type of hand puppet, where the hand fits inside a hollow head and arms, and controls the puppet. The following is for an adult who can place his or her first two fingers inside the head of the puppet, the thumb in one arm, and the last two fingers in the other arm. The head is made from papier-mâché over a hollow tube, which forms the neck. People make the glove puppets for narrative performance work, or simply for the joy of creating something.

You will need

- newspaper and PVA glue
- protective gloves, aprons and table covers as required
- sellotape
- hollow tube for the neck
- two pieces of fabric 30cm x 25cm
- needle and thread (or glue)
- marker pen or fabric pencil
- scissors for cutting cloth
- paint, marker pens or felt for eyes
- wool, netting, material for hair
- fabric scraps for clothes, hats and decoration.

Directions for the head

1. Design the puppet head features (usually based on the individual whose puppet it is).

2. Roll up some newspaper around the end of a tube and tape it in place as a rough head shape to start papering.

3. Either dip or paint the newspaper strips with glue and create three initial layers of papier-mâché. Leave to dry.

4. Create cardboard facial features (cheeks, eyebrows, chin, ears and nose) to fix onto the face with the next three layers of paper. Leave to dry.

5. Cut the cardboard neck length to a size that fits the first two fingers comfortable. The bottom edge can be covered in soft felt or fabric, as some hands are tactile sensitive.

6. Paint the head and eyes when dry and add the hair or fabric hats.

Directions for the body

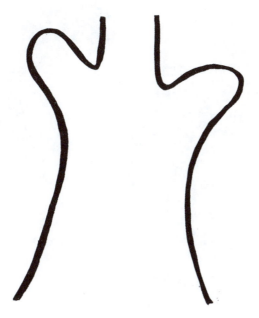

Figure 18 Template shape for glove puppet

1. Make sure the best sides of the main fabric face each other before drawing the glove puppet shape large enough for the hand to spread comfortably.

2. Use the template (Figure 18) as a guide for the basic shape. Note the arm with the lower neck dip is where the thumb fits. Allow an extra 10–15mm around the edge for sewing or gluing.

3. Pin the fabric pieces together before sewing the edges up. Note the bottom of the glove puppet remains open for the hand to get in. The top also remains open.

4. Turn the fabric body inside out, so the right fabric is showing. Also check that the thumb arm is the correct side for whichever hand will be used.

5. Slide the fabric neck over the cardboard neck. Glue in place. The neck can be disguised with scarves, collars and ties (see Figure 19).

6. More material can be cut to create jackets, aprons, cloaks and hats.

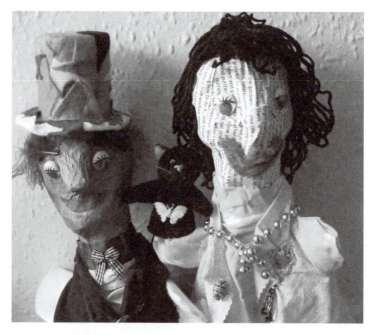

Figure 19 Glove puppets

How to Make a Jointed Rod or Tabletop Puppet

The wooden puppets are popular on our programmes. Sometimes called tabletop puppets, these jointed figures are very flexible. There is a lot more preparation required, but every stage can be made accessible to people with different abilities, concentration spans and understanding. We regularly use papier-mâché heads as described in Appendix 3. The simple rod puppet instructions shown here are developed by Chris King (2012) and use a wooden ball head.

You will need

- head: 50mm wooden ball
- nose and handhold: 8mm dowel x 160mm
- upper body: dressed pine 68mm x 20mm x 75mm
- lower body: dressed pine 43mm x 20mm x 50mm
- arms: 15mm dowel x 35mm (x 4)
- hands: dressed pine 43mm x 20mm x 140mm
- legs: 15mm dowel x 90mm (x 2) and 75mm (x 2)
- feet: dressed pine 43mm x 20mm x 60mm (x 2)

Other materials

- curtain eyes x 20
- sandpaper

- wood glue (white PVA)
- two x 20mm woodscrews
- thin pieces of leather 22mm x 20mm (x 2)
- four small panel pins 10mm (optional)
- strong clear glue
- material for clothes/felt/wool/feathers/paint and paintbrushes or anything else to enhance your puppet's character.

Tools

- drill (with 8mm and 2mm bits)
- bradawl
- wooden mallet
- small wood chisel
- penknife
- tenon saw (or similar)
- long nosed pliers
- screwdriver (to fit the screws you use)
- ruler or tape measure
- pencil
- craft knife or scissors.

Safety

Before working on any piece of wood, make sure it is securely held in a vice or by a clamp to the workbench. Wear appropriate protective gloves and goggles.

Other notes

For the upper body use (dressed) 3 x 1 inch (68 x 20mm) pine (or deal). The lower body, hands and feet are made of (dressed) 2 x 1 inch (43 x 20mm) pine (or deal). All sizes are approximate and may vary depending on the supplier (or what you have lying about in the shed!); a few millimetres won't make much difference to the finished puppet (see Figure 20). Indeed, if you wanted a taller puppet you could extend the legs by a couple of centimetres.

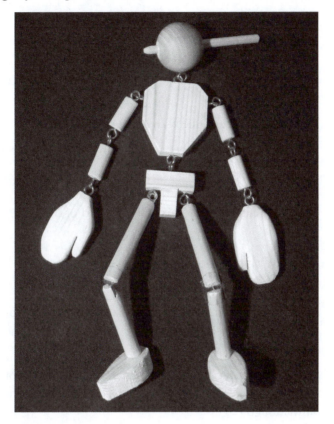

Figure 20 Jointed wooden puppet

Directions for fitting the nose and handhold to the head

1. Using a bradawl, make a guiding hole in the wooden ball.

2. Drill all the way through the head (where you've make the guiding hole).

3. Sand any rough bits and put some wood glue into both ends of the hole.

4. Fit the 8mm dowel into the drilled hole until the nose comes all the way through by about 10mm. The remaining 100mm will be your handhold (this can be shortened to fit your hand if preferred).

5. The dowel may need to be sanded thinner to fit in the hole. Tap it in gently with a wooden mallet.

6. If the dowel becomes too loose, it can be secured by stuffing a mixture of sawdust and wood glue into the joint and leaving it to dry.

7. Wipe off any excess glue with a damp cloth.

8. If desired, the nose can be tapered with coarse sandpaper.

9. When the glue is dry, make another guiding hole with the bradawl halfway between the nose and the handhold. Screw one of the curtain eyes. This will form part of the neck.

Directions for the upper body (68mm across, 75mm down)

1. At the top, measure 10mm across and 10mm down on each side. Cut off these corners using the saw. This creates the puppet's shoulders.

2. At the bottom measure 20mm across and 30mm up on each side. Cut these corners off. This tapers down to the waist. Sand off the rough edges.

3. Using the bradawl, make a small hole in the centre of the top surface and screw in a curtain eye. Open up the curtain eye slightly by using the pliers. This will eventually join up with the eye hook on the head.

4. Do the same at the bottom; this will join up with the lower body.

5. Just below the shoulders make small holes 5mm down and screw in a curtain eye on each side. Open these up with the pliers too. They will be for the arms later on.

Directions for the lower body
(50mm across, 43mm down)

1. From the bottom measure up 25mm and across 15mm on each side. Cut out these sections leaving a T shape. Sand off the rough edges.

2. The legs will hang down from these cutaway sections. At the centre of each one, make a small hole with the bradawl and screw in curtain eyes. These ones can be a bit fiddly so the pliers can be used. Use them again to open up the curtain eyes, ready for the legs.

3. In the centre of the top surface make another small hole and screw in a curtain eye. This will later be used to join with the upper part of the body (which already has an open eye).

Directions for the arms

1. Take two of the 35mm pieces of dowel, make a small guiding hole in both ends of each and screw in four curtain eyes.

2. Open up one of the eyes, slot it through one of the others and pinch it shut again using the pliers. Attach one end to one of the open eyes of the upper body and pinch it shut.

3. Do the same for the other arm.

4. Be careful, the dowel can split if you are too rough. It is a good idea to have a couple of spares just in case. (Or cut off at the split, try again and have shorter arms!)

5. Open up one of the curtain eyes on the end of each arm. These will be for the hands.

Directions for the hands

1. These simple mitten style hands are best done at the same time, while still joined together. That way you get a right and a left hand.

2. Take the 140mm piece of wood and place it lengthways in front of you.

3. On the top corners measure 15mm along and 10mm down and saw out these blocks. On the horizontal cuts, continue for a further 15mm. These bits will form the thumbs.

4. On the bottom corners measure 15mm along and 10mm up. Saw these corners off diagonally. Using the chisel gradually take slivers off each end from about 25mm in tapering down to about half the depth (10mm). The thumbs can be chiselled in the same way, going down in a gradual slope from the end of the cut.

5. Measure along halfway (70mm) and draw a line down. Along the top edge, measure 20mm each way from the centre line and 12mm down. Join these up to form a V shape. Do the same along the bottom of the wood. Cut out these V shapes.

6. Measure 10mm each way from the centre and using the chisel create a slope going back towards the middle to about a depth of 3mm. Do the same on the underneath.

7. Saw down the middle separating the two hands.

8. The wrists can be shaped to approximately 15mm round.

9. Use the chisel (or penknife) to round off any sharp edges. Finally use the sandpaper to smooth them out.

10. Fit a curtain eye to the wrist of each hand. Attach these to the open eyes on the end of the arms and pinch them shut with the pliers.

11. If you have the inclination, a lot of time can be spent carving and sanding the hands and special needle files can be purchased for fine detail.

Directions for alternative hands

1. As the hands are the most time-consuming pieces to carve, here is a simpler alternative (use a strong clear glue).

2. Glue felt onto one side of a piece of thick cardboard (cereal packet will do).

3. When the glue is dry, draw and cut out the two hand shapes.

4. Glue the end of the arm over the cardboard side of the hand by about 25mm.

5. Then glue on another piece of felt over this side of the hand, making sure it will dry tightly around the dowel arm, to keep it firmly in place.

6. When it is dry, cut away the overhanging pieces of felt to tidy it up.

Directions for the legs

1. Mark a line across the middle of one end on each of the pieces of leg dowel. After securing upright in the vice, saw down 10mm on each. Using the chisel (or penknife if you prefer), gradually taper down diagonally from 10mm away to the end where the saw cut is.

2. Fit the leather into the slot on one 90mm piece and one 75mm piece using the strong clear glue. Both the tapered slopes should be on the same side. This should be a tight fit, but if the leather doesn't quite go in the slot, the gap can be widened slightly using sandpaper (which may need to be folded in half).

3. There should be about a 2mm gap between the two sections. This is the knee joint.

4. You can use a small panel pin gently hammered in diagonally from the centre of the tapered slope just to make sure the leather doesn't slip out over time.

5. The leather can be trimmed after the glue has dried using scissors or craft knife.

6. At the end of the shorter piece, drill a hole about 10mm in using the 2mm bit. This pilot hole will be for screwing in the foot later on. At the other end of the longer piece fit a curtain eye. This end will fit to the lower body.

Directions for alternative legs

1. Instead of sawing the slots and gluing in the leather, an alternative is to drill a 2mm hole through both pieces a quarter of the way around and 10mm up.

2. A piece of string can then be threaded through both bits and tied off.

Directions for the feet

1. At one end of the 60mm piece of wood, saw off the back corners to create the back of the foot. Do similarly at the other end to create the toes end (see Figure 21).

2. Using the chisel and sandpaper, round off and smooth all the edges of the foot.

3. Measure in 15mm at the middle. Drill a 2mm pilot hole all the way through. Change to the 8mm bit and drill a countersink hole halfway down (10mm). This is the bottom of the foot.

4. Be careful if using an electric drill, it can go all the way through very easily. If it does, glue in a 10mm piece of 8mm dowel and redrill with the 2mm bit.

5. Attach the foot to a leg with a screw.

6. Again, be careful here. The dowel is quite delicate and can split. Wrapping gaffer tape tightly around the bottom of the leg can help, which may also be left on as socks if you like!

7. Do the same for the other foot and leg.

Directions for joining your puppet together

1. By now you have already joined up some of the parts and the rest is quite straightforward.

2. Fit each of the legs onto the lower body by putting the closed eye over the open eye and pinching it shut with the pliers.

3. Fit the lower body to the upper body in the same way and finally the upper body to the head.

4. The joints of the puppet (where the curtain eyes are attached to each other) have a tendency to move quite erratically. If desired, small strips of material can be wound and tied around the joint to minimise the movement, although if left unchanged the effect can be quite comical.

Finally

1. You may want to make clothes for your puppet.

2. Some people prefer to leave the puppets as natural wood or paint clothes on them.

3. Paint the facial features.

4. Use felt, wool or other material glued on for hair.

5. To use the puppet hold it by the dowel at the back of the head. Your other hand can be used to move an arm or a leg. Slow movements are generally the best.

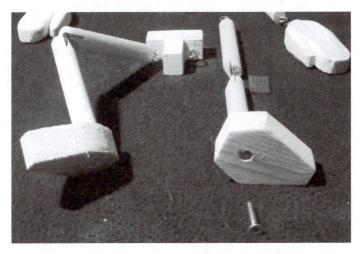

Figure 21 Jointed wooden foot

How to Make a Bird Marionette

There are several approaches to making a bird marionette. This is one of the simpler versions and offers great movement with easy to use controls for any puppeteer. Birds are perfect for dancing, walking with and generally brightening up the place.

You will need

- a long (180cm) feather boa

- two foam balls about 15–20cm diameter

- one wooden ball approximately 8cm diameter sawn in half

- a cross bar (made from two pieces of dowel approximately 30cm in length)

- four pieces of strong thread or nylon fishing wire (plus extra)

- two nails and thin wire

- fabric pieces and felt for eyes, lashes and beak

- additional feathers/jewellery/decoration

- scissors

- strong glue or glue gun

- hammer.

Directions

1. Use various material pieces to create big eyes, beak and lashes on one of the foam balls. The beak could be simply a diamond shape folded in two, or a more substantial stuffed beak.

2. Glue the end of the feather boa to the forehead of the bird head and glue it around the rest of the back and side of the head, leaving the rest hanging from the base of the head to form the neck.

3. Someone can hold the head up as you measure about 30cm of neck length, and securely glue this to the top of the other foam ball. Cut the remaining boa off.

4. Take 60cm of the remaining feather boa, and fold in half to find the middle. With the person holding up the head, make sure the body is in the right position, and glue the fold over the top of the body, just behind the neck. The two legs are now in place.

5. Check the legs dangle evenly. Now glue each end of the leg to the top of the each half of the wooden ball.

6. Attach the strong thread or fishing line, using nails that are hammered and bent to secure in place on the wooden feet.

7. Use the thin wire to create pins that the fishing line can be tied to, and secured with the glue gun into the foam head (at the top near the forehead) and into the body (on top in the middle).

8. Cover the rest of the body with any remaining feather boa or fabric pieces. Small wings are an option.

9. Cut a notch at the end of each dowel, as well as in the centre of the dowels. Glue, nail (and use extra thread) to secure the cross bars at right angles to each other.

10. Someone needs to hold the bird to tie the fishing line onto the dowel notches and adjust the length for the right height (see Figure 22).

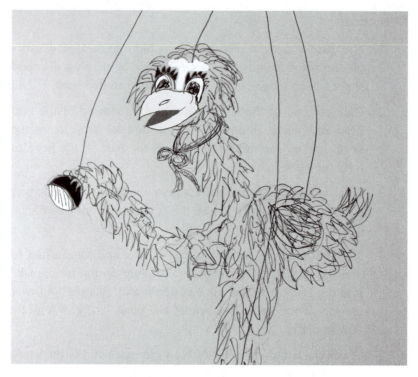

Figure 22 Marionette bird sketch

Contact details

Address
Karrie Marshall
Suite 333
24 Station Square
Inverness
IV1 1LD

Email
karrie@karriemarshall.co.uk

Website
www.karriemarshall.co.uk

Director of Creativity in Care
karrie@creativityincare.org (email)
www.creativityincare.org (website)

References

Abbey, J., De Bellis, A., Piller, N., Esterman, A., *et al.* (2002) *Abbey Pain Scale. Dementia Care Australia Pty Ltd 1998–2002.* Available at www.dementiacareaustralia. com (accessed February 2013).

Afif, A., Hoffmann, D., Becq, G., Guenot, M., Magnin, M. and Mertens, P. (2009) MRI-based definition of a stereotactic two-dimensional template of the human insula. *Journal of Stereotactic and Functional Neurosurgery 87,* 6, 385–394.

Alzheimer's Society (2012) What is fronto-temporal lobe dementia? Available at http://alzheimers.org.uk/site/scripts/documents_info. php?documentID=167 (accessed March 2012).

Andrews, J. (2012) *Arts and dementia.* Paper presented at the Dementia Friendly Arts Symposium, Macrobert Arts Centre; Stirling, October.

Angelou, M. (2013) www.facebook.com/MayaAngelou (accessed February 2013).

Arnoldi, M.J. (1995) *Playing with Time: Art and Performance in Central Mali (Traditional Arts of Africa).* Bloomington, IN: Indiana University Press.

Baines, P. (2007) *Nurturing the Heart: Creativity, Art Therapy and Dementia.* Quality Dementia Care Paper 3. Hawker, ACT: Alzheimer's Australia.

Baldwin, C. (2005) *Storycatcher: Making Sense of Our Lives through the Power and Practice of Story.* Novato, CA: New World Library.

Banerjee, S., Smith, S.C., Lamping, D.L., Harwood, R.H., *et al.* (2006) Quality of life in dementia: More than just cognition. An analysis of associations with quality of life in dementia. *Journal of Neurology, Neurosurgery and Psychiatry 77,* 2, 146–148.

Barbershop Harmony Society (2010) *Health Benefits of Singing.* Barbershop Harmony Society. Available at www.barbershop.org/news-a-events-main/291-health-benefits-of-singing.html (accessed February 2013).

Bateson, M.C. (1993) Composing a life. In C.H. Simpkinson and A.A. Simpkinson (eds) *Sacred Stories: A Celebration of the Power of Story to Transform and Heal.* San Francisco, CA: HarperSanFrancisco.

BBC (2013) *Learn to Sing: Warming Up.* Available at www.bbc.co.uk/sing/ learning/warmingup.shtml (accessed February 2013).

Beresford, M. (1966) *How to Make Puppets and Teach Puppetry*. London: Mills and Boon.

Binder, D.K., Schaller, K. and Clusmann, H. (2007) The seminal contributions of Johann Christian Reil to anatomy, physiology, and psychiatry. *Neurosurgery 61*, 5, 1091–1096.

Black, A.L., Bauer-Wu, S.M., Rushton, C.H. and Halifax, J. (2009) Compassionate silence in the patient–clinician encounter: A contemplative approach. *Journal of Palliative Medicine 12*, 12, 1113–1117.

Blumenthal, E. (2005) *Puppetry: A World History*. New York: Abrams.

Blundall, J. (2012) *The World through Wooden Eyes: The Ideas Store*. Available at www.theworldthroughwoodeneyes.co.uk/history.html (accessed February 2013).

British Medical Journal (2007) Financial cutbacks are hampering the vital support doctors can give carers. Press release by the *British Medical Journal*, July. Available at http://web.bma.org.uk/pressrel.nsf/wlu/SGOY-74ZD9C?OpenDocument&vw=wfmms (accessed February 2013).

Brooker, D. (2004) What is person-centred care in dementia? *Clinical Gerontology 13*, 3, 215–222.

Brooker, D. (2006) *Person Centred Dementia Care: Making Services Better*. London: Jessica Kingsley Publishers.

Browne, W.A.F. (1976) *What Asylums Were, Are and Ought to Be: Being the Substance of 5 Lectures Delivered Before the Managers of the Montrose Royal Lunatic Asylum 1837*. New York: Arno Press Inc.

Bruner, J. (2003) *Making Stories: Law, Literature, Life*. Cambridge, MA: Harvard University Press.

Burkman, K. (1998) *The Stroke Recovery Book*. Omaha, NE: Addicus.

Bussell, J. (1968) *The Pegasus Book of Puppets*. London: Dobson.

Callow, S. (2010) Living with dementia: My mother and I. Talk at St John's Church, Edinburgh.

Chang, B.H., Noonan, A.E. and Tennstedt, S.L. (1998) The role of religion/spirituality in coping with caregiving for disabled elders. *The Gerontologist 38*, 4, 463–470.

Cohen, G.D. (2006a) *The Creativity and Aging Study: The Impact of Professionally Conducted Cultural Programs on Older Adults*. Final Report, April. San Francisco, CA: American Society on Aging.

Cohen, G.D. (2006) Research on creativity and aging: The positive impact of the arts on health and illness. *Generataions 30*, 1, 7–15.

Craick, D.M. (1864) *A Life for a Life*. New York: Carleton. Available at http://openlibrary.org/books/OL24456338M/A_life_for_a_life (accessed February 2013).

Davies, E. and Higginson, I.J. (eds) (2004) *Palliative Care: The Solid Facts*. Geneva: WHO Europe. Available at www.euro.who.int/en/what-we-do/health-topics/environment-and-health/urban-health/publications/2004/palliative-care.-the-solid-facts (accessed February 2013).

Dementia Services Development Centre (DSDC) (2012) *DSDC Virtual Care Home.* Stirling: DSDC, University of Stirling. Available at http://dementia.stir. ac.uk/virtualhome (accessed February 2013).

De Oliveira, C. (2010) Toothbrushing inflammation, and risk of cardiovascular disease: Results from Scottish Health Survey. *British Medical Journal 340,* 2451, 1–6. Available at www.bmj.com/content/340/bmj.c2451 (accessed May 2013).

Department of Health (DOH) (2008) An introduction to personalisation. Available at http://webarchive.nationalarchives.gov.uk/+/www.dh.gov.uk/ en/SocialCare/Socialcarereform/Personalisation/DH_080573 (accessed February 2013).

Dooneief, G., Marder, K., Tang, M.X. and Stern, Y. (1996) The Clinical Dementia Rating Scale: Community-based validation of 'profound' and 'terminal' stages. *Neurology 46,* 6, 1746–1749.

Dowling, J.R. (1995) *Keeping Busy: A Handbook of Activities for Persons with Dementia.* Baltimore, MD: Johns Hopkins University Press.

Dunn, L.A., Rout, U., Carson, J. and Ritter, S.A. (1994) Occupational stress amongst care staff working in nursing homes: An empirical investigation. *Journal of Clinical Nursing 3,* 3, 177–183.

Dyck, P. (2007) Living a quality life with dementia. *Alzheimer's Care Today 8,* 4, 301–303.

Eden, D. (1999) *Energy Medicine.* London: Judy Piatkus.

Emerson, E. (2001) *Challenging Behaviour. Analysis and Intervention in People with Learning Difficulties.* Cambridge: Cambridge University Press.

Erikson, E.H. (1968) *Identity, Youth, and Crisis.* New York: Norton.

Estes, C.P. (1992) *Women Who Run with the Wolves.* London: Ballantine.

Feil, N. (2012) *It is Never Good to Lie to a Person Who Has Dementia.* Cleveland, OH: Validation Training Institute. Available at https://vfvalidation.org/web. php?request=article5 (accessed February 2013).

Finke, C., Esfahani, N.E. and Ploner, C.J. (2012) Preservation of musical memory in an amnesic professional cellist. *Current Biology 22,* 15, R591–R592.

Flood, A. (2009) Classic gags discovered in ancient Roman joke book. *The Guardian,* 13 March. Available at www.guardian.co.uk/books/2009/ mar/13/roman-joke-book-beard (accessed February 2013).

Fontana, D. (1993) *The Secret Language of Symbols.* London: Pavilion.

Fox, K. (1999) The influence of physical activity on mental well-being. *Public Health Nutrition 2,* 3A, 411–418.

Frampton, M. (2003) Experience assessment and management of pain in people with dementia. *Age and Ageing 32,* 3, 248–251.

Friedman, G. (2010) Puppetry workshops for S.E. Asia. Blog on *Puppetry News,* 15 September. Available at http://africanpuppet/blogspot.co.uk/2010/09/ puppetry-workshops-for-se-asia.html (accessed June 2012).

Goffman, E. (1961) *Asylums: Essays on the Social Situation of Mental Patients and Other Inmates.* New York: Anchor.

Golay, L., Schnider, A. and Ptak, R. (2008) Cortical and subcortical anatomy of chronic spatial neglect following vascular damage. *Behavioral and Brain Functions* 4, 43. Available at www.behavioralandbrainfunctions.com/content/4/1/43 (accessed February 2013).

Hall, E.T. (1966) *The Hidden Dimension.* New York: Anchor.

Hannemann, B.T. (2006) Creativity with dementia patients. Can creativity and art stimulate dementia patients positively? *Gerontology 52,* 1, 59–65.

Haslam, C. and Cook, M. (2002) Striking a chord with amnesic patients: Evidence that song facilitates memory. *Neurocase: The Neural Basis of Cognition* 8, 6, 453–465.

Heathcote, D. and Bolton, G. (1995) *Drama for Learning: Dorothy Heathcote's Mantle of the Expert Approach to Education.* Portsmouth, NH: Heinemann.

Henley, J. (2012) The village where people have dementia – and fun. *The Guardian,* 27 August. Available at www.guardian.co.uk/society/2012/aug/27/dementia-village-residents-have-fun (accessed February 2013).

Herr, K. (2002) Pain assessment in cognitively impaired older adults: new strategies and careful observation help pinpoint unspoken pain. *American Journal of Nursing 102,* 12, 65–68.

Herr, K., Bjoro, K. and Decker, S. (2006) Tools for assessment of pain in nonverbal older adults with dementia: a state-of-the-science review. *Journal of Pain and Symptom Management 31,* 2, 170–192. Available at www.sciencedirect.com/science/article/pii/S0885392405006111 (accessed April 2013).

Hicks, E. and Hicks, J. (2004) *Ask and It Is Given.* London: Hay House.

Hogan, S. (2001) *Healing Arts: The History of Art Therapy.* London: Jessica Kingsley Publishers.

Holloway, S.D. (2011) The wounded hero: Explorations in mythology and the performing arts. Excerpt from a paper delivered at the Words and Music Conference, New Orleans, November. Available at www.scribd.com/doc/62460155/The-Wounded-Hero-Explorations-in-Mythology-and-the-Performing-Arts (accessed June 2012).

International Journal of Person-centred Medicine (2012) Geneva Declaration on person-centred care for chronic diseases. *International Journal of Person-Centred Medicine 2,* 2. Available at www.ijpcm.org/index.php/IJPCM/article/view/206 (accessed May 2013).

James, O. (2008) *Contented Dementia: 24-Hour Wraparound Care for Lifelong Well-being.* London: Vermilion.

Jobst, K.A., Shostak, D. and Whitehouse, P.J. (1999) Diseases of meaning, manifestations of health, and metaphor. *Journal of Alternative and Complimentary Medicine 5,* 6, 495–502.

Johnson, J. and Slater, R. (eds) (1993) *Ageing and Later Life.* London: Sage in association with the Open University.

Jones, A. (2013) *Andy Jones Puppet Theatre.* Available at www.andyjonespuppettheatre.com/p/reviews.html (accessed February 2013).

Kane, M. (2012) *My Life Until the End: Dying Well with Dementia.* London: Alzheimer's Society.

Kawashima, R. (2012) Cognitive training for dementia care and prevention. Paper presented at the International Conference of Alzheimer's Disease, London, March.

Kellehear, A. (2009) Dementia and dying: The need for a systematic policy approach. *Critical Social Policy 29*, 1, 146.

Kitwood, T. (1997a) *Dementia Reconsidered: The Person Comes First.* Buckingham: Open University Press.

Kitwood, T. (1997b) *Evaluating Dementia Care: The DCM Method,* 7th edn. Bradford: Bradford Dementia Care Group, University of Bradford.

Kuo, H.K., Yen, C.J., Chang, C.H., Kuo, C.K., Chen, J.H. and Sorond, F. (2005) Relation of C-reactive protein to stroke, cognitive disorders, and depression in the general population: Systematic review and meta-analysis. Taiwan. *Lancet Neurology 4*, 6, 371–380.

Lamura, G., Mnich, E., Nolan, M., Wojszel, B., *et al.* on behalf of the EUROFAMCARE Group (2008) Usage and accessibility of support services for family carers of older people in six European countries: Prevalence findings from the EUROFAMCARE study. *The Gerontologist 48*, 6, 752–771.

Laozi (1986) *The Way of Life According to Lao Tzu.* Translated by Witter Bynner. New York: Perigee Trade.

Laozi (1989) *The Complete Works of Lao Tzu,* revised edn, trans. Hua-Ching Ni. Santa Monica, CA: Seven Star Communications.

Littlechild, B. (1997) *Dealing with Aggression.* Birmingham: Venture Press.

Livesey, L., Morrison, I., Clift, S. and Camic, P. (2012) Benefits of choral singing for social and mental wellbeing: qualitative findings from a cross-national survey of choir members. *Journal of Public Mental Health 11*, 1, 10–26.

Luft, J. (1969) *Of Human Interaction.* Palo Alto, CA: National Press Books.

Lupien, S.J., Schwartz, G., Ng, Y.K., Fiocco, A., *et al.* (2005) The Douglas Hospital Longitudinal Study of Normal and Pathological Aging: Summary of findings. *Journal of Psychiatry and Neuroscience 30*, 5, 328–334.

McKillop, J. and Petrini, C. (2011) Commentary: Communicating with people with dementia. *Annali dell'Istituto Superiore di Sanità (Italy) 27*, 4, 333–336.

MacQuarrie, C.R. (2005) Experiences in early stage Alzheimer's disease: Understanding the paradox of acceptance and denial. *Aging and Mental Health 9*, 5, 430–441.

Manley, K., Hills, V. and Merriot, S. (2011) Person-centred care: Principle of Nursing Practice D. *Nursing Standard 25*, 31, 35–37.

Mares, P. (2003) *Caring for Someone Who is Dying.* London: Age Concern England.

Marshall, K. (1999) *Approaches to Dealing with Challenging Behaviour.* Course Handbook. Inverness: Inverness College, University of the Highlands and Islands.

Marshall, K. (2008) Puppetry for working with people with dementia. Unpublished paper.

Maslow, A.A. (1943) Theory of human motivation. *Psychological Review 50*, 4, 370–396. Available at www.researchhistory.org/2012/06/16/maslows-hierarchy-of-needs (accessed February 2013).

Mehrabian, A. (2009) Interview on *More or Less*. BBC Radio 4. Available at www.presentationworks.me/index.php/2009/11/mehrabian-on-the-myth (accessed February 2013).

Miles, M.F.R. (1994) Art in hospitals: Does it work? A survey of evaluation of arts projects in the NHS. *Journal of the Royal Society of Medicine 87*, 161–163.

Miller, B. (2004) Grandad is an artist! Dementia and the creative mind. Available at www.abc.net.au/rn/allinthemind/stories/2005/1500008.htm (accessed May 2010).

Miracle, V.A. (2007) The power of silence. *Dimensions of Critical Care Nursing 26*, 1, 42. Available at www.nursingcenter.com/lnc/journalarticle?Article_ID=685836 (accessed February 2013).

Montgomery-Smith, C. and Brennan, N. (2003) *Singing for the Brain*. London: Alzheimer's Society.

Museum of Modern Art (MoMA) (2012) *Meet Me: The MoMA Alzheimer's Project*. New York: MoMA. Available at www.moma.org/meetme (accessed February 2013).

Neary, D., Snowden, J.S., Mann, D.M., Northen, B., Goulding, P.J. and Macdermott, N. (1990) Frontal lobe dementia and motor neuron disease. *Journal of Neurology, Neurosurgery, and Psychiatry 53*, 1, 23–32.

Nicholas, M., Barth, C., Obler, C.K., Au, R. and Albert, H.L. (1997) Naming in Normal Aging and Dementia of the Alzheimer's Type. In H. Goodglass and A. Wingfield (eds) *Anomia: Neuroanatomical and Cognitive Correlates*. San Diego, CA: Academic Press.

Nolan, M.R., Davies, S., Brown, J., Keady, J. and Nolan, J. (2004) Beyond 'person-centred' care: A new vision for gerontological nursing. *Journal of Clinical Nursing 13*, 3a, 45–53.

Obraztsov, S. (2001) *My Profession*. Amsterdam: Fredonia.

Office for National Statistics (ONS) (2011) *Deaths: Place of Occurrence and Sex by Underlying Cause and Age Group, England and Wales, Table 12*. In Mortality Statistics: Deaths Registered in 2011 (Series DR), Tables 1–4, 6–14. London: ONS. Available at www.ons.gov.uk/ons/publications/re-reference-tables.html?edition=tcm%3A77-277727 (accessed February 2013).

Otter, E. den (1993) Aids? If only I had known! Puppetry against Aids in Togo. Available at http://elisabethdenotter.nl//site2/sida/sida.html (accessed February 2013).

Papagno, C. (2001) Comprehension of metaphors and idioms in patients with Alzheimer's disease: A longitudinal study. *Brain: A Journal of Neurology 124*, 7, 1450–1460. Available at http://brain.oxfordjournals.org/content/124/7/1450.full (accessed February 2013).

Reisberg, B. and Sclan, S.G. (1992) Functional Assessment Staging (FAST) in Alzheimer's disease: reliability, validity and ordinality. *International Psychogeriatrics 4*, 3, 55–69.

Reisberg, B., Ferris, S.H., de Leon, M.J. and Crook, T. (1982) The Global Deterioration Scale for assessment of primary degenerative dementia. *American Journal of Psychiatry 139*, 9, 1136–1139.

Robinson, G. (2009) *Can Gerry Robinson Fix Dementia Care Homes?* BBC 2 Television, 8 and 15 December. Available at www.bbc.co.uk/programmes/b00pf0s2 (accessed February 2013).

Rockwood, K. (2007) What metaphor for the brain? *Neurology 69*, 20, 1896–1897.

Rogers, C. (1959) A Theory of Therapy, Personality and Interpersonal Relationships as Developed in the Client-Centered Framework. In S. Koch (ed.) *Psychology: A Study of a Science. Volume 3: Formulations of the Person and the Social Context.* New York: McGraw-Hill.

Rogers, C. (2003) *Client-Centered Therapy: Its Current Practice, Implications and Theory.* London: Constable and Robinson.

Roy, C.D. (2002) The art of Burkina Faso. Available at www.uiowa.edu/~africart (accessed May 2012).

Rubin, D.C. (1995) *Memory in Oral Traditions: The Cognitive Psychology of Epic, Ballads, and Counting-out Rhymes.* New York: Oxford University Press.

Salamone, G., Lorenzo, C.D., Mosti, S., Lupo, F., *et al.* (2009) Color discrimination performance in patients with Alzheimer's disease. *Dementia and Geriatric Cognitive Disorders 27*, 6, 501–507.

Schulkind, M., Hennis, L.K. and Rubin, D.C. (1999) Music, emotion, and autobiographical memory: They're playing your song. *Memory and Cognition 27*, 6, 948–955.

Scottish Government (2011) *Standards of Care for Dementia in Scotland: Action to Support the Change Programme, Scotland's National Dementia Strategy.* Available at www.scotland.gov.uk/Publications/2011/05/31085414/6 (accessed February 2013).

Skingley, A. and Bungay, H. (2010) The Silver Song Club Project: Singing to promote the health of older people. *British Journal of Community Nursing 15*, 3, 135–140.

Speaight, G. (1990) *The History of the English Puppet Theatre.* London: Robert Hale Publishers.

Stacy, R., Brittain, K. and Kerr, S. (2002) Singing for health: An exploration of the issues. *Health Education 102*, 4, 156–162.

Staricoff, R.L. (2004) *Arts in Health: A Review of the Medical Literature.* London: Arts Council England.

Stevenson, R.L. (1895) A Penny Plain and Twopence Coloured. In *Memories and Portraits.* New York: Charles Scribner's and Sons.

Stevenson, R.L. (1973) The Land of Counterpane. In I. Opie and P. Opie (eds) *The Oxford Book of Children's Verse.* Oxford: Oxford University Press.

Swaffer, K. (2012) Person-centred care: an insider's view. Paper presented at the International Conference of Alzheimer's Disease, London, March.

Talbot, M. (2011) *Keeping Mum.* London: Hay House.

Tolle, E. (2009) *A New Earth: Awakening to Your Life's Purpose.* London: Penguin.

Tsai, P. and Chang, J.Y. (2004) Assessment of pain in elders with dementia. *MEDSURG Nursing 13*, 6, 364–370.

Van Der Steen, J.T., Pasman, H.R., Ribbe, M.W., Van Der Wal, G. and Onwuteaka-Philipsen, B.D. (2009) Discomfort in dementia patients dying from pneumonia and its relief by antibiotics. *Scandinavian Journal of Infectious Diseases 41*, 2, 143–151.

Vanier, J. (1998) *Becoming Human.* Toronto, ON: House of Anansi Press Inc.

Victoria and Albert Museum (2013) *Make Your Own Toy Theatre.* Available at www.vam.ac.uk/content/articles/m/make-your-own-toy-theatre (accessed February 2013).

Volicer, L. (2010) Caring for patients with terminal Alzheimer's disease. *Canadian Review of Alzheimer's Disease and Other Dementias 13*, 2, 9–14 (May). Available at www.stacommunications.com/customcomm/Back-issue-pages/AD_Review/ad_review/ad2010e.html (accessed May 2013).

Watson, N. (2011) Ephemeral animation: The life and death of objects and puppets. *Puppet Notebook: British UNIMA 19*, 6–8.

Welch, G.F. (2008) *Researching the First Year of the National Singing Programme in England: Baseline Data and an Initial Impact Evaluation.* London: Sing Up Research Group, Institute of Education, University of London.

Whalley, L. (2012) Understanding brain ageing and dementia: A life course approach. Public lecture, University of the Highlands and Islands, Inverness, 28 November. Available at www.uhi.ac.uk/en/media/news/alternative-approach-to-identifying-and-treating-brain-ageing-and-dementia (accessed February 2013).

Williams, P. (1998) *How Stories Heal* (audio CD). Chalvington: Human Givens.

World Health Organization (WH0) (2010) *People-Centred Care in Low- and Middle-Income Countries.* Available at www.personcenteredmedicine.org/docs/geneva2011i.pdf (accessed February 2013).

World Health Organization (WHO) and Alzheimer's Disease International (2012) Dementia Health and Social Care Systems and Workforce. Chapter 4. *Dementia: A Public Health Priority.* Geneva: WHO.

World Health Organization WHOQOL Group (1993) *Measuring Quality of Life: The Development of the World Health Organisation Quality of Life Instrument.* Geneva: WHO.

Wuest, J., Ericson, P.K. and Stern, P.N. (1994) Becoming strangers: The changing family caregiving relationship in Alzheimer's Disease. *Journal of Advanced Nursing 20*, 3, 437–443.

Young, J.G. (1985) What is creativity? *Journal of Creative Behavior 19*, 2, 77–87.

Subject Index

Author Index